EXPLOSIVE
CHILDREN
WITH ADHD

**A NEW APPROACH TO MANAGING ATTENTION
DEFICIT DISORDER IN CHILDREN TO
DISCIPLINE AND EMPOWER YOUR SUPER HERO
TO ACHIEVE SUCCESS AND ACCOMPLISHMENT**

Pansy Bradley

TABLE OF CONTENTS

INTRODUCTION

Every adult hopes to one day become a parent and share in the happiness that comes with raising a child. They talked about how they were going to do things like give their baby a bath, feed them well, and take them to school. The discovery of a disease in a kid might shatter a parent's aspirations for a close bond with their offspring as the youngster matures.

ADHD is a neurological disorder that causes a child to be persistently and inappropriately impulsive, hyperactive, and inattentive. It's the main point of the novel.

The purpose of this publication is to educate you regarding what to check for, how kids with all of this condition feel, and what you can do to help your kid succeed in spite of his or her difficulties.

WHAT IS ADHD (IT'S NOT WHAT YOU IMAGINE)?

Attention Deficit Hyperactivity Disorder is what it sounds like. Basically, it's a health problem that needs to be fixed. Due to differences in brain growth and activity, people with ADHD have trouble paying attention, maintaining focus, and controlling impulsive behaviors. Many aspects of a child's life can suffer when they have this syndrome (ADHD).

Autism spectrum disorder (ASD) is a common neurodevelopmental disease in young children. The process of diagnosis often starts in childhood and lasts far into maturity for many people. Children and teens with ADHD may have trouble paying attention, may not think through the repercussions of their behavior, or may be very energetic.

It's common for kids who have this feature to be very physically active and healthy. Running, playing football, dancing, and other activities that entail considerable physical work are always appealing to them. In situations where they should be discovering new stuffs or working under the supervision of an adult to attain something essential, like school or private tutoring, children with this disorder often act disinterested and uncaring.Young children, especially those between certain ages like three and seven, sometimes have trouble paying attention and behaving correctly. Kids with ADHD do not, however, naturally lose these tendencies as they become older. The signs do not go away and, at times, can be rather severe, making it hard to perform daily tasks or interact with others.

An ADHD child could:

- Have a propensity towards extensive daydreaming.
- Drop the ball and drop something. Many of them fidget or squirm, chat too much, make mistakes, or take unnecessary risks.
- problems with impulse control and waiting one's turn
- conflict with others easily
- do things that require them to use that much effort
- When things get boring, he leaves the room or the classroom so he doesn't have to waste energy standing or sitting still for too long.

Early Years

Symptoms of attention deficit hyperactivity disorder (ADHD), such as a child's increased hyperactivity and impulsiveness, can appear as early as the preschool years. Children's healthcare practitioners may take note of these actions because they can be distracting for the

5

kids and the staff. Teachers may miss red flags if students in issue are easily swayed or pass by without paying attention.

The inattention of a youngster usually becomes more noticeable as they begin elementary school, where focus is increasingly essential.

Younger children are often encouraged to explore their environment and learn via play. Older kids, on the other hand, need to be attentive, patient, and self-controlled as they answer questions quickly and without interruption.

Teenage Years

Adolescents encounter unique challenges due to the increased demands placed on them in terms of autonomy and independence at school and in their personal lives. Imbalances in impulsivity, attentiveness, and self-esteem can lead to unfavorable results such underage drug use, pregnancies, and unsafe driving.

Adolescents with ADHD may experience a worsening of symptoms when they are asked to organize their own time, handle more difficult tasks, and accept responsibility for their own actions.

Adulthood

Some people say their symptoms improve with age, while others say they stay the same. However, adult ADHD is more likely to show itself in an individual who is distracted, inattentive, and too responsive to frustration than in a hyperactive toddler.

Adults can get help for ADHD with medication and behavioral therapy. The accurate diagnosis of ADHD requires the expertise of a healthcare provider who specializes in the disorder.

People with ADHD might display one of three different forms, depending on which set of symptoms is the most prominent. The following are some examples of such expressions:

- **Typically inattentive presentation:**The person has trouble getting started on or carrying out a task, listening attentively to or remembering details, or completing tasks or conversations. In addition, the person has trouble focusing on the finer points of a task. The person has trouble focusing on the details of their regular activities and is quickly distracted.
- **Generally Hyperactive-Impulsive Presentation**: one who speaks quickly and is constantly on the go. It can be difficult to sit still for an extended amount of time (such as during a meal or while completing homework). It's not uncommon to observe toddlers and younger kids always on the move. This individual has trouble controlling their impulsive behaviors and is usually plagued by emotions of restlessness. A person who acts on impulse may rudely

cut off others, steal their belongings, or talk out of turn. It may be difficult for the person to wait one's turn or pay attention to instructions. It's possible that impulsive persons are more prone to damage themselves in accidents.

- **Combined Presentation**: When additional symptoms from the first two categories are present, this is the third possible presentation.

Scientists are trying to determine what causes Attention Deficit Hyperactivity Disorder (ADHD) and what factors enhance a person's chance of acquiring the disorder so that they can create more accurate diagnostic tools and therapies. Few risk factors or causes have been identified for ADHD, but new studies point to a strong genetic component. New studies confirm that ADHD runs in families.

Researchers are investigating not only the genetics of the disease, but also a wide range of other possible risk factors and causes.

- Traumatic Brain Injury
- Pregnant women and children are particularly vulnerable to the harmful consequences of the exposure to environmental risks like lead.
- Use of tobacco and alcoholic beverages during pregnancy
- Premature birth
- Underweight infants

Research does not back up the commonly held notions that poor parenting, too much screen time, or environmental or social factors like poverty or family strife cause ADHD. These are just a few examples of the many things that could make symptoms worse for certain people. Nonetheless, evidence is lacking to support the contention that they are the fundamental causes of ADHD.

In children, ADHD has become the most commonly diagnosed behavioral disorder. A mental health professional, child psychologist, or pediatrician will often make the diagnosis of attention deficit hyperactivity disorder (ADHD) in a kid. Diagnosing attention deficit hyperactivity disorder (ADHD) requires collecting intelligence about the kids development from the child's parents and teachers, observing the child's attitude, and doing psychoeducational testing. ADHD is a syndrome, thus diagnosis includes looking at results from tests that evaluate the patient's health, brain function, and mental state in multiple ways. Some examinations can be used to exclude other conditions, while others can be used to assess knowledge and competence.

Hyperactive habits including fidgeting, impulsive conduct, and inattention are not always indicative of attention deficit hyperactivity disorder in children (ADHD). Symptoms of attention deficit hyperactivity disorder (ADHD) can be caused by a number of different conditions, including anxiety, sadness, learning disabilities, and poor physical health.

Many people with ADHD and similar disorders benefit from early intervention programs. For this reason, it's crucial to employ a tried-and-true procedure for testing and evaluation.

The healthcare professional doing the evaluation must rule out any other possible causes of the patient's observed symptoms before settling on a diagnosis of attention deficit hyperactivity disorder (ADHD).

It's already a difficult situation, but it's believed that anywhere from 60 percent to 100 percentage of kids with ADHD also have comorbid diseases like anxiety, melancholy, behavioral issues, learning difficulties, sleep problems, and drug usage. All of these factors will be taken into account when you craft a treatment plan for your child that is tailored to their unique needs and medical diagnosis.

Environmental Factors

Life changes or stressful situations, such as moving, losing a loved one, dealing with money problems, or even acquiring a new sibling, can bring on symptoms similar to those of attention deficit hyperactivity disorder (ADHD).

Neglect, parental or domestic problems, inconsistent discipline, harassment, abuse, and other complex emergencies can also have significant negative effects on a child's emotional and mental well-being. The resulting distraction, inattention, restlessness, impulsivity, and "acting out" may fool people into thinking the person has attention deficit hyperactivity disorder (ADHD), however these symptoms are not caused by the condition.

Sleep Problems

People's ability to focus is substantially impacted by sleep disruptions. The following are some more things to think about:

- Hyperactivity
- Irritability
- slowness in the sensory, motor, auditory, and visual systems

- mental sluggishness
- Capacity to learn has decreased. Decline in School Achievement

Teenagers who don't get enough sleep are more likely to engage in risky behaviors including cigarettes, drinking alcohol, and using drugs. Drinking and drug use fall into this category. Sleep disturbances can be caused by anything from poor sleep hygiene to medical conditions like sleep apnea and restless legs syndrome, which interfere with the body's natural sleep rhythm. A poor night's sleep is usually brought on by one's own poor sleeping habits.

Disabilities in Mental Health
Anxiety manifests itself in a wide range of ways, some of which are hostility, distractibility, impulsivity, and hyperactivity. Having trouble sitting still and containing fidgeting is a common symptom of anxiety. Poor mental health is a well-documented contributor to the aforementioned sleep issues. All of these signs and symptoms may be related to attention deficit hyperactivity disorder, but they could equally easily be brought on by something else.
Similarly, depression can cause a decline in focus and memory, a lack of desire and the inability to make decisions, as well as a lack of energy, a lack of drive, a lack of organization, poor sleep, and a general feeling of malaise.
Because of the hyperactivity and inattention that characterize ADHD, oppositional defiance and conduct disorder are often misdiagnosed as this disorder.
Anxiety, depression, and disruptive behavior disorders are frequently seen together with ADHD. Each symptom may represent a distinct disorder with its own etiology and treatment requirements, or they may be secondary conditions brought on by the challenges of ADHD.
Attention deficit hyperactivity disorder (ADHD) assessments should not ignore the individual's emotional functioning in favor of focusing on the more obvious disruptive behavioral symptoms.

Obsessive-Compulsive Disorder
More research is needed to determine the precise nature of the connection between OCD and ADHD, which can cause problems with focus and attention. Focusing difficulties may contribute to attention deficit disorder, while difficulty switching gears may stem from obsessive thinking. Tasks may take longer for a person with

OCD to finish because of the time spent on pre-work rituals and ritualistic behaviors.

Abuse of Substances
ADHD has been related to a greater propensity for substance addiction. Substance abuse can cause comparable behavioral symptoms to those of attention deficit hyperactivity disorder (ADHD), and vice versa. Concentration troubles, memory problems, agitation, impatience, babbling, insomnia, irritability, and other behavioral problems can manifest themselves in these situations.

Autism
People on the autism spectrum, regardless of whether they're children or adults, may show signs of attention deficit hyperactivity disorder (ADHD). In stimulating surroundings, they could become excitable, hyperactive, and impulsive; they may have trouble shifting their focus; they may have trouble comprehending social signs and limits; and they may have difficulties interacting socially.
Extreme motor activity and inability to control it are shared features of tic disorders and attention deficit hyperactivity disorder (ADHD). Rapid, identical motions of the face or arms, as well as sounds or phrases, are characteristic of tics. Tics are characterized by involuntary, repetitive movements and vocalizations, in contrast to the fidgeting, motor activity, and chattering that can be indications of attention deficit hyperactivity disorder.

Challenges in Learning and Comprehension
People with learning disabilities often have problems with attention, processing, organization, memory, and learning that are strikingly similar to those of people with attention deficit hyperactivity disorder (ADHD). Academic performance can be hindered by people who have learning difficulties in reading, writing, communication, or mathematics. Disabilities in hearing and seeing also affect one's ability to communicate effectively. Despite the common incidence of ADHD and learning difficulties together, the two conditions are actually separate medical issues.
A child with high intelligence who is not being challenged in school may exhibit ADHD-like behaviors out of frustration. Some examples of such actions include daydreaming, losing patience, and causing a scene. A bad educational fit, a depressing classroom

10

environment, a lackluster curriculum, or inept leadership can all contribute to these issues.

Health Problems

Seizures, thyroid disorders, allergies, iron-deficiency anemia, recurring ear infections, and impairments of hearing or vision can all lead to difficulties focusing, being irritable, acting impulsively, or being hyperactive. Epileptic seizures are one such condition. Adverse medication reactions can mimic the signs of ADHD.

WHAT HAPPENS IN THE CHILD'S MIND WHEN IT "EXPLODES"?

- In general, kids this age are noisy, active, and quick to act on their impulses. The kids climb and run and make a lot of noise while they play. The want to be mobile and explore their environment drives their continual squirming and writhing. To have trouble paying attention, retaining information, and applying knowledge is a common childhood challenge. Being a kid is characterized by these commonalities.
- Normal childhood habits and developmental challenges are exacerbated for a kid with attention-deficit/hyperactivity disorder (ADHD). As a result of the long-lasting, debilitating nature of ADHD symptoms, the child experiences significant challenges in many aspects of life, including academics, social interactions, and family life.
- Children with ADHD are more likely to experience frustration and anxiety. They have issues with executive functioning and can't control their emotions. For instance, it's probable that they'll run into significant difficulties due to:

- Planning \ Prioritizing
- Paying attention to details
- Knowing the Specifics

Their levels of maturity are likewise typically lower. Some kids with ADHD are naturally endearing, gregarious, and popular in school. On the other hand, many people's self-esteem and social connections suffer severely when they struggle with behavioral issues.

Having ADHD can make daily life difficult. All of the following emotions are possible for children to experience.

11

- **Confusion:** A common symptom of this disorder in children is a lack of clarity about their own desires or the best course of action. When people act rashly, they often don't realize they're doing something wrong since they think they're on the right track. Because of this lack of understanding, kids are easily confused when admonished or urged to behave themselves, and may even grow despondent and withdrawn as a result.
- **Disconnection:** A schism is developing between these children and their parents as a result of the harsh methods used to correct their abnormal conduct. When children are disciplined by shouting, spanking, or being grounded, they withdraw and become emotionally distant. You have no idea what this kid is contemplating or what he might do next, thus this situation is quite dangerous.
- **A sense of being disoriented:** Their peculiar behavior also contributes to the feeling of bewilderment. Some parents compare their children too often, which can be especially harmful if the child in question has younger siblings. This could cause them to withdraw from others as they try to make sense of their own feelings of disorientation.
- **A sense of being out of control:** The wildness of their behavior is an expression of their impulsive nature. These children, as was previously indicated, are chronically energetic and seek any available opportunity to release their pent-up energy. If they start wandering all around classroom while the instructor is speaking or take advantage of a breakout session, it could become quite challenging to maintain control over them. It's crucial to keep in mind that such kids are just acting out in ways that other kids might as well, except that they're doing it at the wrong moment and don't know it.
- **Frustration:** Irritation with the erratic behavior of children with ADHD might lead to harsh words or even physical punishment. Imagine how disheartening it could be to act in accordance with your morals only to have everyone else criticize you for it.
- **Restlessness:** Children with this disease have trouble winding down, even when their friends have given up. There's a chance they won't even understand why their friends are so worn out. However, they are a great deal of enjoyment to be around due to their restlessness, which drives them to engage in stimulating activities that also help them expend energies, such as partying and games. Parents can aid their children in attaining some amount of command over their uneasiness by channeling it into a useful activity.

Derogatory and inaccurate stereotypes about children with ADHD diagnoses exist. They may start to think of themselves in negative ways, labeling themselves as "the evil kid," "lazy," or "dumb," yet these are all erroneous assessments.

It's possible that kids with ADHD will struggle in a variety of areas. As a result of their inability to control their overwhelming emotions, individuals often have to face with difficult consequences.

- **School**: Inattentive behaviors can make it difficult to complete schoolwork, and aggressive behaviors can disturb the learning environment and cause disciplinary action.
- **Interactions**: Children with ADHD may have a more difficult time forming and maintaining friendships (ADHD).
- **Development**: Since ADHD is considered a neurodevelopmental problem, its effects on a child's mental and social growth are often delayed.

WHY YOU SHOULD NOT UNDERESTIMATE ADHD

Sometimes parents don't see the connection between these behaviors and ADHD at first. A child may appear to be misbehaving for no apparent reason at all. Some families of young ones with ADHD report feeling helpless, frustrated, or ignored.

When people comment negatively on their child's behavior, it's natural for the parents to feel embarrassed. Because of this, they may begin to wonder if it is somehow related to their own behavior. Children without ADHD have no trouble developing attention, behavioral, and activity regulation skills; those with ADHD have a much harder time doing so.

It will be more challenging to instruct or prevent a child with this condition from acting out as they mature into a teen or an adult because they will have been accustomed to this behavior. Just picture the consequences of treating a kid with this disease as though he or she is "typical," rather than devoting all available resources to helping him or her thrive from the start. Moreover, the youngster would have been singled out for special attention by adults in their life, which would have had a negative impact on their outlook.

Getting a precise solution of attention deficit hyperactivity disorder (ADHD) in adulthood can be challenging due to the fact that symptoms often change between childhood and age. An adult's hyperactivity might reveal itself somewhat frequently than that of a child's or it might take the shape of racing thoughts rather than frantic movements.

Some of the methods used by medical professionals to diagnose adult ADHD are as follows.

- The TOVA is a true test of your attentiveness talents meant to assess how you are able to concentrate on something that is not your first choice. It compares your findings to those of persons who have and don't have ADHD. Individuals with attention issues who are compensating may appear to do well on the Test of Visual Attention Abilities (TOVA), as its results are not always conclusive.
- The Attention and Activity Rating Scale (Conners CAARS) is a tool for diagnosing and assessing adult attention deficit hyperactivity disorder (ADHD) symptoms such inattention, impulsivity, and hyperactivity (CAARS). Used to determine whether or not a person

has ADHD. There is a self-report and witness scale that you and a trusted friend or family member can fill out.

- The Adult ADHD Self-Report Scale (ASRS) is another self-report measure that can help you determine if your symptoms match the DSM diagnostic criteria for ADHD.
- Executive function as measured by the Behavior Rating Inventory–Adult (BRIEF-A): The BRIEF-A is a comprehensive test of your executive functioning, measuring such skills as your ability to focus, prioritize, multitask, and remember information. It accomplishes so by comparing your difficulties to those experienced by persons of a similar age as you.

Parents need a solid understanding of how to parent children with ADHD after they learn their child has the disease. A typical mistake parents make is not recognizing or underestimating their child's disorder and expecting normal behavior. Without adequate care and attention, the youngster may suffer.

The role of the parent is essential in the treatment of ADHD. The manner that parents respond might have a positive or negative effect on their child's ADHD symptoms.

When your child has been diagnosed with ADHD:

- Put out some effort. Learn as much as you can about attention deficit hyperactivity disorder. Follow your child's doctor's orders regarding treatment. Try to make it to all of your therapy appointments. Administer your child's prescribed ADHD medication as directed. Never adjust your dose without your doctor's approval. Your child's medication needs to be stored in a safe, out-of-the-way place.
- Learn how your child will be affected by ADHD. Every single one of these children is special. Examine the difficulties your kid is having to deal with because of ADHD. For some kids, it takes some extra work to learn how to listen and focus. People should learn to slow down relatively frequently. Talk to your kid's therapist about what you can do to help them improve their skills at home.
- Focus on instructing your kid one thing at a time. Don't try to do too much all at once. Try to keep things low-key at first. Just think on one thing. Say "thank you" to your kid for making an effort.
- Parental involvement at your child's school is encouraged. Talk to your kid's teacher to figure out if he or she needs a 504 or an IEP. Schedule regular conferences with your child's teachers to discuss how they are doing in class. Please work with your child's educator to ensure his or her success.

- To raise awareness and support, band together with others. If you have ADHD and want to learn more about current treatments and other resources, consider joining CHADD or another support organization.
- In order to diagnose ADHD. Inattention deficiency hyperactivity disorder runs in many families. Some families with children who have Attention Deficit Hyperactivity Disorder (ADHD) have mom and dad or other close family members who are uninformed of the disease. Successful parenting is possible once parents with ADHD have been diagnosed and treated.
- Intentional and caring discipline. Find out what kinds of discipline help children with ADHD and what kinds of discipline make the illness worse. The therapist your child is seeing should be able to give you some guidance on how to deal with the situation. Children with ADHD may be easily hurt. Instead of being harsh, try correcting their conduct in a nice and supportive manner.
- Bring your expectations into focus. Before leaving the house, have a conversation with your kid about the behavior you expect from them. Put more energy into teaching your child what to do rather than correcting them when they do something wrong.
- Talk about it. You should talk to your kid about ADHD. Help kids understand that they aren't alone in dealing with ADHD symptoms, and that there are ways to cope.
- Invest extra time into your daily routine to bond with one another. Set aside some time, even if it is only a few minutes, to spend with your kid, talking, doing something fun and relaxing that you both enjoy, and giving your undivided attention to them. Celebrate productive efforts. Don't go overboard with compliments, but do acknowledge good behavior. Encourage your youngster to wait their turn by saying something such as, "You're enjoying each other's company so beautifully."
- The love you have for your kid is the most crucial factor. Children with ADHD might worry that they are bad people because of their actions. Your child's sense of self-worth may be protected if you model these traits of tolerance, acceptance, and patience. It's important to show your kid that you value and respect who they are and what they bring to the table. Strengthen your child's resilience by keeping up a positive and loving relationship with them.

You may be advised to try out behavioral treatment options before commencing any pharmaceuticals. Behavioral therapy can help people with ADHD develop new ways of handling stressful situations. You might also help them learn more appropriate methods for expressing their feelings.

Behavioral modification parenting classes are also offered. They will be able to deal with their child's behavior with this knowledge. Additionally, it could help in the creation of methods for dealing with the illness.

For kids under 6, behavioral treatment is the gold standard and is generally initiated without medication. Children above the age of 6 may have a better chance of benefiting from a combination of behavioral therapy and medication.

Cognitive behavioral therapy, parental or marital counseling, meeting with an ADHD coach, and using classroom management techniques are all potential treatment options for adults and children with ADHD. A support group can be an emotional lifeline for people who have ADHD and their dear ones.

With the earlier-mentioned measures in place, youngsters with this disorder can be monitored and cared for more effectively, leading to improved control of the disorder and greater calm for the kid. The child's life will be more centered and well-rounded as a result of this. Therefore, the kid will have a healthy outlook, and he or she will be able to socialize with others and act normally.

HOW TO RECOGNIZE THE EXACT VARIANT OF YOUR CHILD'S DISORDER

One simple test is not available for diagnosing attention deficit hyperactivity disorder (ADHD). Usually, signs and symptoms appear before a child becomes 7 years old. However, the symptoms of ADHD are shared with a number of other disorders. Your doctor may do a variety of tests to check out potential causes like stress, anxiety, and sleep issues before arriving at a diagnosis.

At least six of the nine core symptoms of ADHD are required for a diagnosis. To be diagnosed with mixed ADHD, at least six symptoms of attention problems and hyperactive-impulsive behavior must be present. At least six months of noisy and pervasive behavior is required.

Symptoms must also have been present before the age of 12 and include a record of inattention, hyperactivity-impulsivity, or both. Both the classroom and the family area should have them readily available.

In addition, the symptoms have to get in the way of daily life. As an added bonus, these symptoms cannot be explained by any other known mental disorder. Identifying a youngster with ADD or ADHD is a multi-step process (ADHD). Read this article to find out more about the detection and diagnosis of ADHD. Insomnia, anxiety, depression, and even some forms of learning disability may share symptoms with attention deficit hyperactivity disorder (ADHD), and there is currently no reliable diagnostic test for the problem.

Talking to a doctor about whether or not a child's symptoms are consistent with attention deficit hyperactivity disorder (ADHD) is the first step in making a diagnosis.

Depending on the circumstances, it may be possible to identify only one subtype of ADHD at the time of initial diagnosis. Keep in mind that your symptoms may change over time. An updated evaluation in the context of this new data may be helpful for adults.

Each subtype of ADHD is associated with its own unique collection of signs and symptoms. Symptoms of attention deficit hyperactivity disorder include fidgetiness and impulsivity (ADHD).

Examples of such behaviors include the following:
- Inattentiveness: Inattention manifests itself through a lack of concentration and haphazard actions.

- Hyperactivity: Hyperactivity manifests as in restlessness, chattiness, fidgeting, and an inability to concentrate.
- Impulsivity: being impulsive and making snap judgments.

It's typical for people to respond differently to a similar stimulus because of their own unique characteristics. As an example, there are clear gender differences in how boys and girls handle these situations. It's usual to generalize that boys are more outgoing and attentive while ladies are more introverted and distracted.

Depending on how you're experiencing such symptoms, a diagnosis of ADHD may be made.

Inattentive Type

This form of ADHD is characterized less by impulsivity and hyperactivity than by a general lack of focus. To maintain self-control or initiative under such conditions might be challenging. However, these are not the most obvious signs of inattentive ADHD.

People who regularly miss class tend to be the ones that forget things, become bored easily, have trouble focusing, follow directions, don't engage, move slowly, appear to daydream, take in knowledge more slowly and less precisely than others, and struggle to follow even the simplest of tasks.

Inattentive ADHD affects a disproportionate number of women.

Hyperactive-Impulsive Type

Characteristics of this kind of ADHD include impulsivity and hyperactivity. This form also includes symptoms of inattention, but they are milder than in the other forms.

People who have a tendency for impulsivity or hyperactivity often exhibit the following:

a type of movement that displays restlessness, fidgeting, or wriggling

Act aggressively, skip their turn, fail to consider the effects of their actions, respond inquiries and make comments too rapidly, and generally be "on the go" and unable to stay still for long.

It's possible that children with hyperactive-impulsive ADHD will disrupt the classroom. They pose a risk to the educational experience of themselves and their peers. Hyperactivity/impulsivity is more commonly diagnosed in males than females.

Combined Type

Your symptoms suggest a combination type, rather than inattention or hyperactivity/impulsiveness alone. Rather, symptoms from both categories are manifested.

Both those with and without ADHD can exhibit bouts of acute inattention and impulsivity. Those who suffer from ADHD, however, endure a more severe type of this. This increasingly common behavior has a negative effect on your capacity to carry out the responsibilities of daily life in the home, in the class, in the workplace, and in your interpersonal relationships.

More boys than females suffer from the combined form of ADHD. The most common symptom in young children is a state of restless activity.

Depending on how your symptoms progress, you might find that your diagnosis of ADHD changes over time. A person's struggles with attention deficit hyperactivity disorder (ADHD) may continue throughout their lives. With the assistance of remedies like medication, people can have a higher standard of living.

AN OVERVIEW OF THE POSSIBLE CAUSES OF ADHD

No one has yet pinpointed a cause for ADHD. Scientists suspect a number of variables play a role in determining who develops ADHD. Factors such as genetics, the environment, prenatal infection, and underlying health conditions have all been proposed as possible causes.

Still, many things can go wrong to cause ADHD, and we'll go over some of those here.

The etiology of attention deficit hyperactivity disorder (ADHD) remains unknown. There are a number of risk factors that can affect whether or not someone develops attention deficit hyperactivity disorder (ADHD).

- Genetics
- Chemicals and pollutants in the environment
- Prenatal drug and alcohol use disorders
- Birth Before It's Due

Genetics

After coming into contact with an ADHD youngster, one's natural inclination is to question if the disorder runs in the family. Hyperactivity/attention deficit hyperactivity disorder (ADD/ADHD) has strong hereditary components. It is thought that genetics play a role in over 70 percent of ADD/ADHD cases.

It's not a guarantee that an ADHD parent would automatically pass the disorder on to their child, despite the significant genetic relationship between the two. This is because the likelihood that a child may acquire ADHD depends on a nuanced interaction between hereditary and environmental factors. It is possible for a child to inherit ADHD genes and never show symptoms of the illness.

It's possible that more than one gene contributes to ADHD in families. It is likely that many genes, in addition to environmental influences, contribute to the development of attention deficit hyperactivity disorder (ADHD).

ADHD is a disorder that affects both sexes equally. In other words, attention deficit hyperactivity disorder (ADHD) is not limited to males and is not necessarily passed down through the paternal line. Some people mistakenly believe that only dads can have attention deficit hyperactivity disorder (ADHD) and that a kid cannot develop the condition unless neither of his relatives has. It's completely false.

Although ADHD is more commonly diagnosed in boys than girls, it is important to keep in mind that the illness can affect anyone.

Susceptibility Genes

Due to its high inheritance, research into the genes that cause attention deficit hyperactivity disorder (ADHD) has intensified. Investigating common DNA variation has been the cornerstone of molecular genetic studies of ADHD up until this point. According to the common disease-common variation hypothesis, this is also true for other chronic conditions. Candidate gene techniques, which presume a disorder's pathogenesis to explore, were used first. As of late, this has been researched by 'hypothesis-free' GWAS, in which the rates of hundreds of single nucleotide polymorphisms (SNPs) throughout the genome are matched between cases and controls. More and more people are starting to wonder if rare genetic changes might play a part in the development of attention deficit hyperactivity disorder.

The strongest evidence linking ADD/ADHD is found in variations of the dopamine D4 receptor (DRD4) gene (ADHD). Exon III of the gene contains a functional polymorphism (varying number tandem repeat—VNTR) that has been studied extensively because of the receptor's ability to bind dopamine and norepinephrine. This polymorphism, such as the seven-repeat allele, has been linked to ADHD in a number of meta-analyses. Recent meta-analysis shows statistically meaningful link with moderately small effect size despite extensive heterogeneity between studies.

The DRD5 gene, which encodes a different type of dopamine receptor, has also been consistently implicated. Many meta-analyses have found a genetic marker called a microsatellite to be associated with attention deficit hyperactivity disorder (ADHD), even though evidence suggests substantial variability among studies.

The dopamine transporter gene (DAT1) was at first thought to be the most likely candidate gene for attention deficit hyperactivity disorder (ADHD) because it is willing to take responsibility for inhibiting the release of dopamine in the presynaptic cleft, which is inhibited by stimulants, and also because the DAT1 knockout mouse exhibits hyperactivity and deficits in inhibitory behavior. The most often investigated variation (a VNTR in the untranslated region (UTR) region of the gene) was discovered to have a 480-bp allele, and considerable evidence of relationship was observed with other polymorphisms in the same gene in the most recent meta-analysis. There was a correlation between this evidence and a higher probability of getting sick. Multiple variants in this gene enhance the risk of ADHD, which may account for the reported significant heterogeneity despite the fact that these relationships have not been broadly replicated. The large variation could also be the result of a gene-environment relationship in between UTR VNTR and prenatal variables like maternal alcohol intake or smoking.

The catechol O-methyltransferase (COMT) gene, which is important for catalyzing the breakdown of dopamine, has also been the subject of extensive study. The valine-to-methionine switch has been the focus of numerous genetic studies because of a functional difference in the gene. The enzyme's function is altered by the change. The results of meta-analyses and pooled analyses failed to show a correlation between the investigated factors and ADHD. Research, however, indicate that COMT may act as a modifier of the ADHD phenotype instead of an independent risk factor for the disorder. Patients with ADHD were found to be more likely to engage in antisocial conduct if they carried the COMT Val/Val genotype (which is linked to higher enzyme activity). Two independent populations confirmed this result when their data were merged for analysis. Numerous other investigations have replicated the connection findings, suggesting that impaired social understanding mediates the link to antisocial conduct. Those who need a citation: Those who need a citation: This association can be said to be unique to anti - social behaviour in persons with ADHD because it hasn't been detected in the absence of ADHD and other psychiatric conditions.

Illnesses and Injuries

Infections of the meninges and brain (encephalitis) can cause cognitive and attention problems.

It has been found that a few people develop attention deficit hyperactivity disorder (ADHD) symptoms as a result of brain injury carried on by an early brain injury, trauma, or other blockage of normal brain development.

For up to a decade after a non-catastrophic traumatic brain injury, children have a higher likelihood of acquiring attention deficit hyperactivity disorder (ADHD).

Toxins and Diet

Certain environmental exposures appear to be important to the ADHD phenotype; they include organic pollutants like those contained in pesticides, polychlorinated biphenyls (PCBs), and lead.

These may be harmful to the brain's cognitive and nervous systems, both of which are known to play a role in ADHD.

The relationships among organophosphate pesticide exposure and ADD/ADHD were studied using measurements of pesticide levels in umbilical cord plasma and prenatal and postnatal (childhood) urine organophosphate metabolites (ADHD).

PCBs are a class of man-made chemicals that were formerly manufactured in large quantities and are now widely accepted to be detrimental to human health. Research into the impact of PCB exposure on neurobehavioral outcomes similar to those affected by ADHD has been conducted in both humans and animals. Evidence of deficits in working memory, reaction suppression, and cognitive flexibility has been discovered in these investigations. Newer prospective research has shown a dose-response association between prenatal PCB exposure and ADHD-like behavior in middle childhood. It was also established that there was a statistically significant relationship between the two variables. Cognitive flexibility, alertness, and awareness are the most consistently impaired aspects of executive processing and attention in both human and animal studies of lead exposure. Evidence from multiple research suggests that even trace amounts of lead may have a role in attention deficit hyperactivity disorder (ADHD), although this is insufficient to draw any firm conclusions about cause and effect. As such, more study is needed to determine the relative role of pesticides and PCBs as drivers of ADHD.

Many different food components, including glucose, synthetic food colourants, zinc, iron, magnesium, and omega-3 fatty acids, have been studied in relation to ADHD symptoms. Magnesium and omega-3 fatty acids are two other components of the diet that have been the subject of research. There is no solid evidence to date that suggests diet plays a major role in the onset of ADHD. Symptom relief by dietary modification is a separate issue. Overall, the trials investigating the relationship between nutrition and ADHD are not very helpful because of their small sample sizes, sensitive outcome measures, and inconsistent intervention techniques. Thus, there is a lack of proof that changing a child's diet can help with ADHD symptoms. However, a limited exclusion diet dependent on foods that had either high IgG or low IgG suggests that it may have a positive impact on the symptoms of ADHD and oppositional defiant disorder, according to the results of a recent randomized controlled experiment.

Psychological Adversity

Poor parental knowledge, low socioeconomic status, poverty, harassment or peer victimization, harsh parenting, abuse, and unrest within the family have all been associated to ADHD. So far, however, research approaches have fallen short of proving that they are indisputable triggers for attention deficit hyperactivity disorder. Longitudinal and intervention studies both suggest that children with ADHD are more likely to have negative mother-son and peer interactions, for example. This is in contrast to the findings of child conduct problems and antisocial behavior among children, where several study methods, including therapeutic interventions, have repeatedly pointed to unfavorable social and family conditions as the causal factor. Conversely, in persons with a genetic predisposition to ADHD, psychosocial variables may modify the condition's expression. Comorbidities, like conduct disorder, depressive symptoms, and functional impairment, may be influenced by these variables.

Extreme deprivation in one's formative years stands out as a prominent exception to this rule. In a study of British adoptees from Romania, researchers saw a pattern of impulsivity and restlessness. Still out in the air is whether or not the same pattern of deficits appears in response to hardship that is less severe than that experienced.

Chemicals And Pollutants In The Environment

A higher rate of attention deficit hyperactivity disorder has been linked to exposure to certain environmental contaminants in childhood (ADHD). Exposure to even low amounts of lead can result in behavioral problems like impulsivity and inability to sit still. Lead was also found in high concentrations in gasoline and in homes that had been painted before 1978.

ADHD may have a number of factors beyond just genetics. It can be challenging to ascertain whether environmental risk factors actually have a causal role in ADHD, despite the fact that several have been related to the disorder. Symptoms or problems in the kid or parent (negative causation, for instance, peer rejection, familial adversity, low socioeconomic position, or head damage) or unmeasured variables, which can include genetic factors, may account for many reported correlations. Even if there is an increase in the number of persons with ADHD being identified, analyses of past patterns have not shown an increase in the condition's prevalence among the general populace over time. There is currently insufficient data from cross-national studies to conclude that the awareness of ADHD is lower in any particular country.

statistics on childhood behavioral disorders, on the other hand, indicate that the incidence of these difficulties has risen in the past 50 years and differs geographically. These results provide credence to the theory that multiple, relatively insignificant environmental influences contribute to the development of ADHD. The combined impact of these elements is fairly stable throughout historical contexts and national boundaries. Some of these adverse effects on health may be attenuated by genetic factors (gene-environment interaction). Epigenetic processes that are tissue-specific allow environmental dangers to alter gene function. For example, research on animals have demonstrated the deleterious effects of early rearing on stress responses via such systems, and that these physiological alterations can be passed down down the generations.

Prenatal Drug and Alcohol Use Disorders

The development of attention deficit hyperactivity disorder (ADHD) in a kid may be influenced by the health and actions of the pregnant mother or father. Deficiencies in both nutrition and infection during pregnancy have been associated to an increase in the prevalence of attention deficit hyperactivity disorder (ADHD) in offspring. Prenatal substance abuse also appears to raise the risk of ADHD in children.

Cigarette smoking during pregnancy has been related to an increased risk of having a child with attention deficit hyperactivity disorder (ADHD). Children exposed to secondhand smoke are at a higher risk for developing attention deficit hyperactivity disorder. The research did uncover a correlation between cigarette smoking and ADD/ADHD, but it could not confirm causation.

Some studies have found that children whose mothers drank alcohol during pregnancy were more likely to be diagnosed with ADD or ADHD as adults. The likelihood that a child may acquire attention deficit hyperactivity disorder (ADHD) was found to increase dramatically among those whose parents regularly drank four or more alcoholic beverages on any given occasion, or who drank lightly to moderately on a regular basis.

Clinical and epidemiological findings support a link between prenatal exposure to maternal cigarette smoking (as measured by mother accounts and urine cotinine levels) and the development of ADHD in the offspring. Despite the biological plausibility that smoking impacts physiological systems that may produce risks related to the etiology of ADHD, it is challenging to appropriately adjust for social and genetic confounds in observational methods. This is due to the documented effects of smoking on the body's physiology. New evidence reveals that genetic and family factors may explain the association between ADHD and low birth weight. This is in contrast to the previous conclusion that a smaller weight gain is not correlated with an increased risk of ADHD due to genetics and the environment.

High maternal alcohol consumption during pregnancy can result in fetal alcohol syndrome. A youngster with this disorder may have trouble focusing and be overly active. It's common knowledge that alcohol can cause birth defects. However, there is no solid proof that even occasional mild drinking during pregnancy increases a child's risk of developing ADHD. There is also inconsistency in the results when looking at the connections between prenatal drug use and offspring outcomes.

There is evidence to suggest that mothers who experience high levels of stress throughout their pregnancies may have children who display ADHD symptoms. New evidence suggests, however, that this may be a reflection of maternal-fetal gene-environment association rather than a causal factor in ADHD (but not in antisocial behavior or anxiety). Despite reports linking mother stress during pregnancy with ADHD in children, this is still the case. In conclusion, with the exception of the severe phenotype of fetal alcohol syndrome, there is still inconclusive evidence that maternal smoking, substance abuse, and stress during pregnancy play a large causative role in ADHD. Despite the fact that there are a number of circumstances that are unfavorable to the results for other potential kids, this holds true.

However, studies have found that maternal alcohol use does not raise the incidence of ADHD in offspring. The findings of this study showed that the offspring of women who drank while pregnant were much more likely to exhibit some ADHD symptoms, however these symptoms might not have been severe enough to fulfill diagnostic criteria.

- Given behaviors are typical of people of a certain age. It's possible for some people to have below-average cognitive abilities while others don't. This is due to the fact that people's brains do not grow at the same rate. A youngster of 10 years of age, for instance, might only have the abilities of an 8-year-old child rather than those of children of the same age. Therefore, the issue is not that your child's

ADHD grows worse as they get older; rather, the issue is that their talents are not developing in tandem with their age.

- Disruptive behaviors (such as finishing a task on time) become much more challenging as the complexity of the tasks demanded of an individual with ADHD increases with age and conditions, such as increasing requirements in school. The demands placed on an individual with ADHD increase in complexity as they age and face new challenges, but the condition itself does not "grow worse." For example, if the kid hands in their assignment late, they run the danger of getting a lower grade. Some other common types of issues are:

- **Undertaking new challenges without enough support**: School is full of unexpected and more harder challenges. The academic demands placed on a youngster increase in complexity as he or she advances through the school grades. A child may have to do things like study multiple chapters of a history book or write lengthy reports. Children with less capacity to meet demands may find it difficult to keep up with the reading, vocabulary, and math requirements, in addition to the societal needs of engaging with peers. If parents and educators do not provide students with ADHD with sufficient support, the condition may worsen.

- **Often, children are punished for actions they can't control**: Parents and educators are more prone to reprimand and chastise children with ADHD. Peers may mock them due to their poor performance in class and inability to keep information from day to day. In addition, some kids with ADHD might not understand how to communicate socially with their peers. Managers can give adults consequences for not getting their work done, and in some situations, family members can do the same if they don't stay organized or focus on their tasks until they're done.

- **Additional problems with thinking, emotions, and behavior**: Anxiety and depression are common mental complaints among those with ADHD. The likelihood that a child will have any kind of issue increases by 62%. Adults with ADHD are six times as likely to suffer from a comorbid condition. Those with ADHD are also more likely to abuse drugs and alcohol.

- **Stress**: A person with ADHD already has a lot on their plate, and there are plenty of things that can cause them worry. Some instances of such events are severe illness, domestic violence, the end of a marriage, the loss of a job, or the death of a close relative or friend.

In conclusion, there is strong evidence that genetic variables play a role in causing ADHD; nevertheless, non-inherited variables, that mostly include environmental consequences and unpredictable events (especially de novo genetic alterations), also play a crucial role in the illness. No one factor has been found as a definitive basis of attention deficit hyperactivity disorder (ADHD), and the health conditions that have been discovered thus far appear to be umbrella terms. Risk factors include chromosomal microdeletions (like VCFS), large and unique CNVs, extremely low weight, and preterm delivery appear to affect a wide range of neurodevelopmental and psychiatric features. Genetic hazards certainly include multiple similar gene variants with a low effect magnitude, but these have not yet been identified. As the price of DNA sequencing continues to drop, finding uncommon variants in the human genome will certainly become a priority. Common structural variations (CNVs) and other uncommon mutations with high risk profiles will likely fall into this category.

Even while we have made great strides in genetics, there is still a lot we don't know about the threats posed by the environment. Multiple techniques are needed to identify the causal causes in ADHD, despite the fact that many factors have been implicated. 45 The strongest evidence comes from associations between ADHD/ADHD-like symptoms and uncommon but extremely trying circumstances. Premature delivery, low birth weight, fetal alcohol syndrome, and early-life institutionalization are all examples of these kinds of adversity. Less is known about the risk factors that affect ADHD's outcomes. One exception is the association among COMT and antisocial conduct in children with ADHD. This correlation has been extensively researched and supports the idea that ADHD-related behavioral issues may stem from unique causes.

The existing data suggests that those with a family history of ADHD or other neurological or learning issues, as well as those who have been introduced to the environmental challenges mentioned above, are at a higher risk of developing the disorder themselves. This data helps to a limited extent in identifying populations at increased risk. However, neither the environmental nor the genetic risk factors may be employed as diagnostic tools or biomarkers for attention deficit hyperactivity disorder (ADHD). Currently, the pathophysiology of ADHD is poorly understood, but it is hoped that future advances in the discovery of ADHD risk variables and routes will allow for better diagnosis and treatment.

HOW TO ENSURE ADHD DOESN'T LEAD TO OTHER FORMS OF DISTRESS SUCH AS ANXIETY, DEPRESSION E.T.C

Diagnosticians for ADHD typically come from the mental health and primary care fields. A psychiatric evaluation entails discussing your vital signs with your caregivers and having them complete a battery of tests and questionnaires regarding your health, your family's health, your academic and home life, and other factors. To ensure no other health problems are present, a doctor may suggest an assessment.

ADHD isn't the only disorder whose symptoms could be caused by anything else. Mood problems, anxiety, substance misuse, brain trauma, thyroid abnormalities, and medications like steroids can all hinder a person's ability to learn. Co-occurring mental health diseases include oppositional defiant disorder (ODD), conduct disorder (CD), anxiety disorders, and intellectual difficulties. A comprehensive psychiatric evaluation is thus essential. Regular imaging and blood tests are not adequate for diagnosing ADHD. To evaluate the severity of a patient's symptoms, clinicians may use computerized tests or refer them for extra psychological testing (such as neuropsychological or psychoeducational testing).

Tics

Tics are characterized by involuntary, recurrent movements. They show up in a variety of illnesses, ADD being only one of them.

It's not uncommon for adults to miss children's tics, even when they're serious enough to require intervention. They are sometimes overt and irritating.

If your child has attention deficit hyperactivity disorder (ADHD), they may engage in unusual habits like blinking or wrinkling their nose repeatedly (ADHD).

Perhaps a teacher was the first one to observe the tics. Many kids feel this way because of the many ways in which education can amplify their existing feelings.

- fatigue\stress\anxiety/excitement

A youngster with attention deficit hyperactivity disorder (ADHD) may appear to be tic-prone because of the disorder. However, it is much more likely that it is the outcome of an untreated tic disorder.

Tic disorders are not included in the diagnostic category of attention deficit hyperactivity disorder, despite their prevalence (ADHD). There is also no evidence that they are associated with ADD or

ADHD. Because of this, some children with ADHD don't exhibit any tic symptoms at all. When a person has both attention deficit hyperactivity disorder (ADHD) and a tic disorder, the ADHD symptoms will often appear first. As a result, an early assessment of ADHD may be made, even if that condition is not the root problem of the tics.

One crucial neurobiological feature shared by TS, ADHD, and OCD is disinhibition, or the failure to regulate socially inappropriate conduct.

Lack of inhibition typically presents as impulsivity in people with TS. Individuals with TS often have difficulties maintaining focus, much like those with attention deficit hyperactivity disorder (ADHD). The presence or absence of these symptoms allows for the diagnosis of TS or ADHD.

Like people with OCD, some people with TS feel driven to engage in rituals in an attempt to stifle disruptive, unwanted ideas. Tics must be performed in a specific manner or for a predetermined amount of repetitions in order to satisfy an urge or sensation.

A child with ADHD who tics may have the disorder portrayed as the cause. However, it is far more probable that it is caused by a tic disorder that has not been addressed.

Tic disorders are not included in the diagnostic category of attention deficit hyperactivity disorder, despite their prevalence (ADHD). There is also no evidence that they are associated with ADD or ADHD. Because of this, some children with ADHD don't exhibit any tic symptoms at all. When a person has both attention deficit hyperactivity disorder (ADHD) and a tic disorder, the ADHD symptoms will often appear first. As a result, an early assessment of ADHD may be made, even if that condition is not the primary reason of the tics.

One crucial neurobiological feature shared by TS, ADHD, and OCD is disinhibition, or the inability to control socially inappropriate conduct.

Lack of inhibition typically presents as impulsivity in people with TS. Individuals with TS often have difficulties maintaining focus, much like those with attention deficit hyperactivity disorder (ADHD). The presence or absence of these symptoms allows for the diagnosis of TS or ADHD.

Like people with OCD, some people with TS feel driven to engage in rituals in an attempt to stifle disruptive, unwanted ideas. Tics must be performed in a specific manner or for a predetermined amount of repetitions in order to satisfy an urge or sensation.

Whereas most instances of ADHD are diagnosed in children and teenagers, the condition often continues into adulthood. Tourette's syndrome can, however, go away on its own. That may imply that certain people with ADHD will be able to outgrow their tic symptoms. Tics are common in children and adults, but there are therapies that can help reduce their severity. Treatment options mostly consist on behavioral therapy and medicines.

Patients can learn to manage and reduce their tics with the help of treatments like behavioral therapy. One of the most praised forms of treatment is the ability to reverse negative patterns of behavior. It has been shown that only the act of verbally identifying tics might increase awareness of them in the person doing so. To help them break their tic habit for good, they try something fresh. Putting one's hands on one's hips may help someone with a tic who feels the need to scratch at their skin resist the urge.

Comprehensive behavioral intervention for tics (CBIT) has also been found to be effective. CBIT therapists treat tics by teaching their patients to avoid situations that bring on tics. The next step is to alter their environment in a way that reduces or eliminates potential tics triggers.

It may be recommended that a child avoid noisy, busy places for a while if they find that the child's tics worsen in certain settings.

The environment could also be altered to make tics less noticeable. In order to make room for a student with tics, teachers may suggest changing furniture or relocating desks.

Depression

People with both ADHD and depression may receive a dual diagnosis.

ADHD adults have a higher suicide rate and suicide attempt rate than the general adult population. Studies show that 30% of people with ADHD may experience significant depression or another mood disorder at a certain point in their lives.

People who have both ADHD and depression tend to have more severe symptoms of either illness than those who have either ADHD or depression alone. People who suffer from both ADHD and MDD should be especially vigilant in keeping their depression under control while they are also receiving therapy for their hyperactivity.

ADHD sufferers have a fourfold increased risk of developing major depression. Hyperactive/impulsive people are at a higher risk of suicide than the general population.

When untreated, ADHD has been linked to depressive episodes. Secondary depression is a condition experienced by some persons with ADHD as a product of their daily struggles with negative emotions.

People who have attention deficit hyperactivity disorder (ADHD) often struggle with poor self-esteem and a negative perception of themselves as a result of the many challenges that come with living with the disorder, such as difficulties in school, interpersonal relationships, work, and the ability to focus on and complete tasks requiring executive function.

For this reason, it may be important to ensure that ADHD is properly managed and treated in order to lessen the effects of depression. One study found that just around a quarter of adults with ADHD were receiving adequate care. As an added precaution against social isolation and feelings of otherness, people with ADHD must be given respect, care, and affection.

Anxiety

Anxiety and ADHD are distinct conditions, yet they often occur together in individuals. A similar number of adults suffer from both ADHD and anxiety disorders. If this describes you, rest assured that anxiety and ADHD symptoms can improve with treatment.

Anxiety can amplify the effects of several ADHD symptoms, like irritability and trouble focusing. Anxiety disorders, on the other hand, feature their own distinct cluster of symptoms, including Persistent Anxiety About Diverse Problems, Nervousness, Stress Fatigue, and Sleep Disturbances.

Anxiety disorders require consistent, excessive worrying. It's a mental illness that can disrupt your life in many ways: at home, at work, and in your community.

Co-morbidity, the occurrence of ADHD in addition to another medical condition, is common. It's possible that those with ADHD are hardwired to experience higher anxiety.

The symptoms of any mental health disorder, if left undiagnosed and untreated, would undoubtedly worsen and may even trigger further problems, such as anxiety.

Behavior risk taking is more common in people with ADHD. Unforeseen implications, such as relationship, familial, and financial challenges, as well as difficulties at work, may result from these dangers.

People with ADHD are typically more impulsive than the general population. Someone with ADHD could take action before fully considering the repercussions, leading to a mountain of stress and anxiety-inducing issues.

As a matter of fact, alcohol abuse has been linked specifically to attention deficit hyperactivity disorder. Alcoholism increases the risk for the development of anxiety disorders.

When deciding between ADHD treatment and anxiety treatment, your doctor will likely take into account which problem affects you more. If your ADHD therapy also makes you feel less anxious, you may not need to take anxiety medication as well.

Treatment for attention deficit hyperactivity disorder can have the following effects:

- Don't worry so much.
- Learn to focus more in order to better organize your time.
- Strengthen your resolve to deal with your anxiety.

Learning disabilities

Despite the fact that ADHD can exacerbate existing learning disabilities, it is not a handicap in and of itself. People with ADHD may struggle academically because of signs including inattention and impulsivity. The inattentiveness and impulsiveness that characterize ADHD are not, in and of themselves, a learning disability (LD), but they do make it challenging for persons with ADHD to learn.

A "disorder in one or several of the fundamental mental factors involved in comprehending or using speech, spoken or written," impacting one's ability to hear, understand, speak, copy, write, spell, or compute. Problems with perception include dyslexia and the gradual onset of aphasia.

Experts agree that neurological issues have a contribution to learning impairments by making it more difficult to take in, absorb, and communicate new information. Another possible cause is genetics.

Learning difficulties and academic skill acquisition difficulties significantly below age level, manifesting in the early school years and lasting at least 6 months, and not attributable to cognitive disabilities, developmental disorders, neurological disorders, or motor disorders characterize neurodevelopmental disorder.

Given that both ADHD and learning difficulties are neurodevelopmental conditions, the fact that people often suffer from both at the same time is not surprising. Researchers have varied their estimates of the frequency of such co-occurrence, although most place it between 30 and 50 percent. To what extent does this double whammy play a role?

- people with both ADHD and LDs have difficulties with working memories and processing speed; This correlation between ADHD and LDs can be attributed to inattentive symptoms rather than hyperactive-impulsive ones;
- There appears to be a complex genetic basis for both ADD/ADHD and reading issues.

- Cognitive and behavioral explanations alone are insufficient to account for the correlation between ADHD and LDs.

TRIGGER FACTORS AND HOW TO AVOID THEM

Identifying the specific type of ADHD you are experiencing is an important first step in developing an effective treatment plan. As was said before, there are actually three different types of ADHD. People who tend to appear inattentive often struggle to maintain order in their personal lives, complete activities, focus on details, and remain focused during conversations. Restlessness, inability to remain still, excessive or inappropriate speech, and impulsivity exhibited through behaviors such as seeking for objects without considering, interrupting others, or engaging in unsafe conduct are all hallmarks of the hyperactive-inattentive subtype of the disease. If a person exhibits symptoms of both forms of ADHD, they are referred to as having a mixed presentation.

While there is currently no treatment capable of completely eliminating symptoms of attention deficit hyperactivity disorder (ADHD), it is possible to keep symptoms under control. In order to begin managing your ADHD, you must first learn to recognize the triggers.

Overstimulation, device use, poor sleep hygiene, and high levels of stress are common triggers for ADHD symptoms.

You can take preventative measures for your child's attention deficit hyperactivity disorder if you understand what triggers his or her episodes.

Stress

Stress has been linked to the onset or exacerbation of ADHD symptoms. Additionally, stress is a possible daily companion for many with ADHD. This could have a number of potential origins.

Evidence suggests that stress has an effect on the same part of the brain as attention deficit hyperactivity disorder (ADHD), the prefrontal cortex.

Additionally, an ADHD child has difficulty focusing and filtering out distractions. Fear increases as a direct consequence. Deadlines, procrastination, and neglect can all contribute to an already difficult situation by causing unnecessary anxiety.

Unmanaged stress may amplify the negative effects of ADHD. Consider the stressed-out behavior of a child with this disease. Is their normal level of energy higher than average? Do you sense that they're less able to concentrate than usual?

Daily stress management is essential, so try out new techniques like meditation or deep breathing, and take more breaks from work.

Poor Sleep

A common symptom of Attention Deficit Hyperactivity Disorder in children is difficulty falling or staying asleep. Many symptoms and signs of attention deficit hyperactive disorder can be attributed to a lack of sleep (ADHD).

Anybody can have their thoughts slow down from lack of sleep. Lack of sleep can increase or even cause the following difficulties when managing ADHD:

- Negligence and forgetfulness
- a lack of energy and the inability to restrain oneself
- inattentional lapses
- The rate of response slowed as performance did.
- Focusing Issues
- challenges in comprehension
- hyperactivity

Young people with attention deficit hyperactivity disorder (ADHD) may benefit from a regular sleep schedule of 7 hours or more every night.

Food and additives

It is still unknown whether or not one's diet might affect ADHD symptoms.

The body and brain may benefit from the ingestion of meals high in nutrients such proteins and omega-3 fatty acids, minerals like calcium, magnesium, zinc, and vitamins B, C, and D. This may lead to a decrease in ADHD symptoms.

The consumption of the following item has been linked to a rise in ADHD symptoms.

- Sugary foods and refined carbs
- A variety of salty treats
- glucose and starch
- Foods that are heavy in saturated fat and caffeine, as well as those that have been chemically preserved with ingredients like sodium benzoate and monosodium glutamate (MSG),

More research is needed to determine whether or not particular foods or food additives may contribute to or aggravate the symptoms of attention deficit hyperactivity disorder disorder (ADHD). Learn which foods are aggravating your symptoms and which are helping you feel better. By keeping track of how food and produce affect you after eating them, you may eliminate the ones that don't agree with you.

When you've already come to terms with the fact that you suffer from ADHD, you can begin making the adjustments to your daily life that will allow you to establish healthy routines and steer clear of circumstances that set off your symptoms. Keep in mind that psychotherapy and counseling are the two most successful treatments for ADHD. Adults with ADD/ADHD frequently undergo CBT (CBT). Working with a specialist to identify and manage your individual triggers is a great first step in developing an effective treatment plan.

Children with ADHD can benefit from a number of lifestyle changes, including adopting a healthy, balanced diet and eliminating caffeine. Several nutrients, such as calcium, magnesium, fatty acids, proteins, and vitamin B, have been demonstrated to reduce the severity of ADHD symptoms in human studies. According to WebMD, having a shopping list can help you stay focused on buying nutritious foods. Regular exercise is a fantastic way to control the symptoms of Attention Deficit Hyperactivity Disorder (ADHD), whether you have the hyperactive-inattentive or mixed versions of the disorder. People with any type of ADHD can benefit from regular exercise since it improves health and lowers stress levels. Avoiding electrical gadgets and other forms of uv light in bed will help you get better sleep. For children with attention deficit hyperactivity disorder (ADHD) who have problems falling or staying asleep, a weighted blanket can be a welcome stress reliever and sleep aid. If you're worried that you might have ADHD, it's best to be checked out.

Overstimulation

Overstimulation of the senses is a common sign of ADD/ADHD (ADHD). In cases of sensory overload, you may experience the following symptoms:

- Sight: Brilliant, bright, or flashing lights can cause visual overstimulation.
- Scent: Strong or unpleasant odors might be a trigger for certain people.
- Sound: Music, fireworks, or a group of people all talking at once might be overstimulating.
- Tongue: Sensational overload can occur when one is exposed to extremes of flavor, temperature, or texture.

The physical contact could be too light, too forceful, too rough, too unanticipated, or too sudden, leading to overstimulation.

The brain's capacity to make meaning of its environment is impaired by excessive stimulation. Being in a very stimulating setting, like one with a loud TV, an awful café, or a crowded mall, might lead to overstimulation.

To minimize overstimulation, it's best to keep the environment free of the kind of things that could bring it on. However, there are other instances where evasion is futile. In cases like this, the following techniques may prove helpful:

- Ahead of time, prepare yourself for the barrage of stimuli that will greet you.
- Put on noise-cancelling headphones, earplugs, or sunglasses.
- A break should be taken whenever the need arises.
- Make some space for yourself where you may go to think things out and relax.
- Avoid spending too much time in places where you'll be bombarded with stimuli.

Technology

ADHD symptoms may be exacerbated by the continual stimulation of electronic devices such as mobile phones, tvs, and the Internet. There is some evidence that television can increase the symptoms of attention deficit hyperactivity disorder (ADHD), although the extent to which it does so remains controversial.

Loud noises and fast-paced images do not trigger attention deficit hyperactivity disorder. An someone with ADHD may find it extremely challenging to concentrate when looking at a bright screen.

Because you are not glued to a computer for hours at a time, you are more inclined to get out and move around, which is great for relieving stress. Put a time limit on how much time you spend daily glued to the TV or online.

Here are some things to keep in mind;

- Only during adult-supervised family video conversations should infants and toddlers under 18 months old be exposed to media.
- Between the ages of eighteen months as well as 2 years old, television use should be restricted to educational content viewed alongside a caregiver or a parent.
- Children in elementary school and younger should limit their screen usage to one hour throughout the week and a maximum of three hours on the weekends.

- Getting kids aged 6 and up to reduce their device use in lieu of other activities is still important.

Individuals, or those attempting to help a child, can employ the following methods for dealing with triggers that bring on symptoms:

Eating a healthy balanced diet

Due to the fact that various mineral shortages have been connected to the beginning of symptoms, proper nutrition takes on added importance for persons with ADHD. Oils, such as healthy fats, like olive oil, and proteins obtained from a wide range of plant sources, such as vegetables, fruits, grains, and legumes, are examples of nutrients that fit in a healthy, well-balanced diet.

You should consult a doctor if you notice that your child's appetite has decreased after taking a stimulant. If the child's weight continues to drop, the doctor may suggest adjusting the drug's dosage or transferring to a new prescription.

Avoiding trigger foods

Avoiding foods with artificial food colorings may be a good idea if you want to keep your child's hyperactivity under control.

Although it is possible that certain food additives contribute to the development of ADHD symptoms in children, it is not always possible to determine which ones. It's feasible that retaining a food journal and noting any negative reactions could aid parents and guardians in identifying out which foods are generating problems.

In order to diagnose which foods are triggering an immune response, an elimination diet might be performed. You resist providing the child any meal that may provoke your signs for a few weeks. To identify the problematic foods, you gradually reintegrate them.

Limiting screen time

For children with ADHD, some parents have found that reducing their screen time has helped. In addition, it may improve the standard of your night's sleep.

Children under the age of five should not spend upwards of one hour in front of a screen per day, according to experts. Children ages 6 and up should have strict and consistent limits put on their screen usage by their parents and caregivers.

If you are a parent who is looking for ways to limit your child's screen time, you may find some of the recommendations helpful:
- Planning out the child's TV time in relation to other activities
- If you really must have the television on while you work, either turn it off or turn it on mute.
- Putting down the phone and other devices at the table
- restricting electronic device use in the bedroom before sleep

Exercising
Recent studies have shown that physical activity can help reduce the symptoms of attention deficit hyperactivity disorder (ADHD). The improvement of several indicators of mental acuity have been linked to increased physical activity. The children will display faster processing times and improved inhibition.

Mindful meditation
Mindfulness meditation involves paying attention to one's present-moment experiences, both bodily and environmental. Since one of the main goals of mindfulness practice is to train oneself to focus on certain things, it has been speculated that meditative practices with a strong emphasis on mindfulness could help reduce symptoms of ADD and ADHD in both children and adults.

Making use of task planning strategies
Children who struggle with executive functioning may benefit from strategies that help them get their bearings and take on challenging new tasks. Several of them are as follows;
- Making routine tasks as interesting as possible
- task-splitting to create more manageable chunks of work
- Time management techniques that involve employing alarms and watches as motivators
- Using diaries for record-keeping and reflection making a conscious effort to focus on the task at hand

UNDERSTANDING "HIDDEN MESSAGE" BEHIND EACH CHILD'S OUTBURST AND HOW TO MINIMIZE IT

The inability to focus or sit quietly for further than a few moments is a common symptom of attention deficit hyperactivity disorder (ADHD) in children. As a result, they struggle to focus and take in new data as rapidly or correctly as their peers. To make matters more challenging for their caretakers, this may impair their capacity to comprehend the outcomes of their activities.

For many kids with ADD/ADHD, self-control is a major issue. Conversely, people's natural inclination is to react emotionally to every given situation. A child requires the capacity to pause, reflect on what has happened and how they feel about it, think about the possible outcomes of their actions, and then use this data to determine whether or not to engage in the behavior again.

Many youngsters who have ADHD struggle to connect their thoughts and behaviors. When a lot of things happen at once, they don't take the time to consider their options and often make hasty decisions as a result.

This may explain why children with ADHD appear to have greater difficulty than their typically developing peers in general when it comes to learning from their mistakes.

Another sign of a problem with working memory is difficulty "seeing what lies ahead." Therefore, it may be difficult for a child to remember information that could guide their behavior.

Children with ADHD may also have delayed development of their internal voice, which helps them "talk" to themselves about what they should do, weigh their options, and regulate their behavior.

Your child who analyzes and reacts spontaneously can benefit from your cues, reminders, rewards, and coaching if you implement them at the point of accomplishment, when they are required to self-regulate their behavior in order to meet of the situation.

You can help your child "put on the brakes" or "stop and think" before reacting by giving them instant feedback about their behaviour and attitude, such as pointing out, bolstering, and satisfying the desired behavior, and giving mild reprimands and rerouting to help them get back on path when they start acting inappropriately.

The ability to reflect on one's own actions and gain insight into one's own strengths and faults is enhanced via such training and upbringing. As your child grows in self-awareness and sensitivity, you'll see an improvement in his or her capacity to make connections between behaviors and their outcomes.

It is crucial to be consistent when imposing sanctions. It is crucial that timely and consistent feedback receive adequate attention. Your child ought to be able to spot the rules without any difficulty. Using these techniques, you may make sure your child always has the same routine.

In general, there are a number of strategies that can be implemented to lessen the intensity of these kids' tantrums. These young people just want to be accepted for who they are without having to continuously defend their every action. In most cases, parents are too quick to judge their children for engaging in out-of-character behavior.

Some of the activities that can be performed regularly to reduce these kids' tantrums are listed below.

Always Pay Attention To Them

Young children respond very well to encouragement and praise. Indeed, they require it. They want it so badly that they will occasionally resort to dishonesty to obtain it. Giving your child your undivided attention is a great way to motivate and reward them.

It's possible that spending time with an ADHD youngster might be exhausting and frustrating, so naturally, they lose their listener's attention over time. They want to be acknowledged but do so at inconvenient times or in bothersome ways, and in the midst of everyone else's wants, they do not always receive it.

At least three times a week, you should set aside an hour to play with your child alone. Take part in their activities on their own terms and you'll fit right in. Comply with their instructions. We recommend beginning with "More of our playtime should be spent in tandem, in my opinion. Pick an activity for yourself to accomplish for the following fifteen to twenty minutes.

As a result, you and the kid will gain a deeper understanding of one another. If a youngster is engaging in small misbehavior that you wish to discourage, try ignoring him or her for a few seconds. If a child is being extremely disobedient, the best thing to say is, "OK. Our unique fun was over after this. We can proceed once you're ready to act in a decent manner.

Praise The Child Constantly

Young children respond very well to encouragement and praise. Indeed, they require it. They want it so badly that they will

43

occasionally resort to dishonesty to obtain it. Giving your child your undivided attention is a great way to motivate and reward them.

It's possible that spending time with an ADHD youngster might be exhausting and frustrating, so naturally, they lose their listener's attention over time. They want to be acknowledged but do so at inconvenient times or in bothersome ways, and in the midst of everyone else's wants, they do not always receive it.

At least three times a week, you should set aside an hour to play with your child alone. Take part in their activities on their own terms and you'll fit right in. Comply with their instructions. We recommend beginning with "More of our playtime should be spent in tandem, in my opinion. Pick an activity for yourself to accomplish for the following fifteen to twenty minutes.

As a result, you and the kid will gain a deeper understanding of one another. If a youngster is engaging in small misbehavior that you wish to discourage, try ignoring him or her for a few seconds. If a child is being extremely disobedient, the best thing to say is, "OK. Our unique fun was over after this. We can proceed once you're ready to act in a decent manner.

Make Use of Rewards

Oftentimes, the homework we give our children is boring and routine. A game on the iPad or a marathon of Netflix is far more appealing to them at this time. We certainly can't say we blame them. Everyone desires freedom to pursue their own interests. How should we teach our kids to be good people when they don't yet have the capacity to do things entirely out of kindness?

Your medicine will taste better if you add some sugar to it. Motivating your youngster to follow your instructions and do what you say can be made easier with the use of rewards and other incentives. Because they encourage the actions you would like to see more of, rewards are of particular benefit when some actions don't appear to have any clear "payoff" (i.e., chores).

Furthermore, there is no need to stress; rewards might be something other than money or physical goods. Rewards can be anything from quality time with a parent to more screen time to being allowed to stay out late to going on a special outing without having to do any of the usual chores. Motivators can take any form the sender sees fit.

The essence of any incentive system is the creation of a coin currency that can be traded for the completion of predetermined tasks. This rewards system can be implemented using anything from a simple ledger to a chart with stickers or poker chips.

Put away the dishes and get a sticker; wash the car and get four stickers; and so on. For example, avoiding having to do one job for 10 stickers, a movie with mom for 20 stickers, and staying awake 30 minutes later for 30 stickers all require explicit guidance on what habits will be compensated, how much will be paid for each activity, and what prizes can be redeemed.

After two weeks, you may introduce penalties (such as taking away stickers or coins for certain actions), but bear in mind that the objective of a bonus system is to encourage habits through motivations, so make sure the benefits still greatly outweigh the penalties!

Effective Instructions

Attention deficit hyperactivity disorder (ADHD) is a prevalent cause of classroom disruption for kids. It's not uncommon for folks to be too distracted by something else or forget what you just said.

- **Gain the Child's attention:** You shouldn't scream from the other room. Make eye contact.
- **Keep it short, clear, and simple**: Provide only a single or maximum of two stages simultaneously.
- **Ensure time is clearly stated**: Specify the timeframes within which you expect this to be completed.
- **Ask for confirmation**: If you have any doubts about whether or not they listened, have them repeat it back to you.
- **Be respectful**: Practice compassion. Matter-of-fact. Please excuse yourself if you've interrupted.

After taking these measures, you can feel comfortable that they didn't miss your request or simply forget. This means that individuals will be held accountable for their choices and must live with the results.

Consistent Consequences

Consequences that are consistently bad are necessary to teach kids valuable lessons. While there is always a consequence for our actions, not all of them are positive. By experiencing the consequences of their own terrible decisions in a reasonable, consistent, and plain manner, children understand the importance of compliance and respect.

Children are skilled manipulators who can make us appear like the most miserable parents if we don't yield in (or, given the persistence of a child's tantrum, give up!). But if we don't follow through with the consequences we set, the problem takes on a new dimension: They are encouraged to persist in their defiance, regardless of the method they choose (ignorance, raving, yelling, pestering, tantrums, etc.). What a recursive loop!

Three considerations to bear in mind while imposing sanctions:

- When you make a threat, back it up with action. You should never make a threat.
- The punishment must fit the crime.
- Immediate consequences are required.

Finding the source of challenging behavior in our kids with special needs is our obligation as parents, and often the child's reaction to our actions is the real problem. Children may begin to question their own worth if they are criticized for being difficult. They've given in to shame. It's possible that the internal conflict that results from having one's conduct questioned can be enough to spur a person to make positive changes. However, it typically causes stress and, less obviously, rage. In contrast, maintaining contact with our children is essential but not always simple. They need to feel heard and valued in order to feel comfortable speaking up. As money is the exchange rate of our economy, so is connection the value of our relationships.

There has been no progress in treating ADHD. This has been a great learning opportunity for both us and our children. Not to mention, tactics are irrelevant. Everyone should try to have an optimistic outlook. The purpose is not to develop habits. What's at risk is the state of our hearts. In addition, children who experience a great deal of genuine love and connection are less likely to feel guilt, are more likely to be physically and emotionally well, and are more likely to succeed in their academic and social endeavors.

Those with ADHD frequently seek out the company of others with the condition. A vibrant conversation may be maintained since their energies are complementary and they share a common desire for similar stimulation. Wow, that's amazing. By pushing each other to achieve more, though, they can quickly find themselves in over their heads. Children with ADHD are at a higher risk of engaging in potentially harmful activities, such as drug usage, sexual experimentation, and other types of self-exploration, according to research. So, monitor your children but don't suffocate them. Friendships between adults whose kids have ADHD can be very helpful.

THE HIDDEN STRENGTHS OF ADHD CHILDREN AND HOW TO UNLEASH THEM

In many ways, people with ADHD are the driving forces behind society's most progressive ideas and innovations (attention deficit hyperactivity disorder). People with ADHD are blessed with an abundance of brilliant ideas and the perseverance to follow them through. Focusing on one's strengths can help people with ADHD achieve greater success and fulfillment in life.

It's common to focus on the difficulties of living with attention deficit hyperactivity disorder. In order to effectively manage and support persons with attention challenges, it is necessary to have a firm grasp of the issues involved. When thinking about your child's ADHD, it's crucial to look outside the proverbial box and take into account the whole child.

Some kids who have trouble focusing also have issues with their own sense of worth. There can be several causes for this. Young people often have a firm grasp on the ways in which they fall short when compared to their contemporaries, but they may be fewer aware of the manner in which they succeed. In addition, it's a fact that kids with ADHD seem to be more likely to have a record of receiving punishment for doing things the right way and more prone to repeat actions that adults view as bad.

Acknowledge and validate your child's disappointment and anger. Take use of your child's ADHD strengths. Step one is helping them recognize the value in these characteristics.

The excellent news is that kids with ADHD can (with the right kind of support and direction) learn to harness and improve their innate abilities, strengths, and skills so that they can go on to have fulfilling and successful lives. They could be endowed with exceptional features and turn out to be quite helpful.

Imagination and Creativity

People with ADHD tend to be extremely creative, ingenious, and imaginative. They are masters of "out of the box" thinking and can keep several thoughts in their heads at once.

People with these characteristics often see things in new ways. It's common for their originality to stem from either in-depth knowledge of the topic at hand or a genuine passion for it.

Rather than being a detriment, your child's creativity should be embraced and nurtured while he or she deals with ADHD. A child's perseverance in the face of difficulty is greatly enhanced by parental patience and encouragement. Is it possible for you to guide your child in using their ADHD strengths to learn more about something that really interests them?

Here are some suggestions to foster your child's creative thinking:

- Activity in the performance arts, especially the arts of speech and song
- "Participating in a Musical Performance"
- Putting down roots and building a foundation
- Clever ways of expressing oneself: artwork
- Solutions and categorization techniques (mathematics, patterns)
- Coding (computing) (computing)

Children with ADHD may have difficulty with time management and multitasking. It's crucial for parents to have patience. If they are given a framework and guidance in these areas, kids will have greater room to experiment and grow their creativity.

Impulsivity and Spontaneity

Individuals with ADHD frequently:

Someone with this personality could be more likely to gamble than they need to. Establishing and maintaining reasonable restrictions and goals is essential before beginning any project because lack of fear in the face of probable success or failure can improve the likelihood of either.

the absence of self-doubt or an interior critic that may otherwise act as a brake on creative thinking. Although these traits may cause problems in social situations, impulsivity often proves to be an asset in other areas of life.

To give only one illustration:

- Usually, this means trusting your instincts.
- Put your dreams into action. It makes it easier to make snap judgments that will move you closer to your goals.
- As a result of your preparedness, you will be in a better position to take advantage of opportunities as they present themselves.
- Being able to act on the spur of the moment opens up opportunities for personal development and growth that would not exist otherwise.

You can benefit from a little bit of spontaneity if:

- Amplify Your Skills
- Create a sense of safety
- Intensify Your Productivity

- In the face of adversity, train yourself to think and behave more fluidly and flexibly.
- Promote and motivate your own development.

Most children will try your patience and push your buttons. Some people may struggle to accept limits, even if such limits are intended for their own safety. Patience and understanding are musts. Your child's safety depends on you being firm with your rules and limits.

Energy and Enthusiasm

Some children with ADHD have almost endless supplies of energy. An abundance of stamina is a valuable trait in many contexts. Because of this, kids may develop a feeling of "superpowers," "ability," and a "anything-is-possible" attitude. They can find that this attribute is one of their biggest helps in managing their ADHD.

Your child's limitless energy can be put to good use in a number of educational and enriching activities.

Here are a few illustrations:

- **Trampolining**: Your memory improves and your stress levels drop. Positive mood-altering hormones are secreted. Facilitates better stability and coordination. Facilitates the development of a solid core muscle structure.
- **Scouts/Guides**: In these kind of situations, one can improve their interaction, cooperation, physical fitness, sympathy, and goal-setting abilities. It is ingrained in young minds that there is value in stretching one's boundaries and taking chances.
- **Visiting museums**: They shouldn't have any further inquiries after reading this. You might think about taking your kid to an interactive museum where they can learn while playing. They get plenty of practice using their motor skills.
- **Building things**: This may entail proceeding as planned or taking an alternative tack. Everything your child does, from figuring out solutions to problems to making decisions to working toward a goal, will need the use of their intellect.
- **Swimming**: This is an excellent way to boost your strength and endurance.

Resilience and Perseverance

To keep up with the demands of everyday life, several children with ADHD have to work harder than their neurotypical peers. Eventually, they grow more determined than ever to achieve their goals. In comparison to their neurotypical peers, adults with ADHD appear to be more resilient.

The resilience of children has to be acknowledged, encouraged, and applauded. Some examples of a child's resilience that can be ascribed to ADHD are shown below.

- Exhibits a genuine interest in and enjoyment of academic work.
- Finds useful approaches to problems
- Proves self-starting, assertive, and enthused.
- Self-reliant; competent to get things done on their own

Hyperfocus

The brain of someone with ADHD is truly one of a kind. Hyperfocus is a common trait among those who suffer from this condition. A child that has ADHD may get so fixated on one thing that they lose track of their surroundings.

The parents may call their child's name repeatedly without any response. They are afraid that their child's mind will entirely shut down. They could get so involved in their work that they forget to eat or tidy up.

Maintaining hyperfocus is a juggling act. In other cases, the youngster with ADHD won't even realize how much stress and frustration they're generating for those around them. They are thus able to devote their full attention to a pursuit that actually thrills and motivates them.

Hyperfocus: Examples and Advantages

- A school assignment may require your child's full attention.
- Kids can become experts at anything they put their minds to and work at for enough time and effort, whether it's an equipment, a computer game, or a sport.
- Reading aloud to your child is a fantastic approach to improve their reading skills and comprehension.
- Taking an active interest in anything that could benefit them intellectually, professionally, or otherwise in the future.

Acquired organizational skills

Irregular behavior and memory loss when trying to follow instructions. Young people with ADD/ADHD often learn strategies to improve their memory and organizational skills (lists, reminders, etc.).There are many success stories about persons with ADHD who attribute their achievements to their extraordinary ability to stay organized.

Great Conversationalist

Those with ADHD have a never-ending supply of novel ideas floating around in their heads.

Conversations sparked by that bottomless source of ideas are guaranteed to be interesting, enlightening, and one-of-a-kind.

Risk Takers

Symptoms of ADHD, such as a desire for novelty and an inability to plan ahead, may lure some people to the challenges and rewards of starting their own business. In the professional sector, people who struggle with ADHD and hyperactivity may benefit from prioritizing efficiency above precision.

Using the five tenets of self-control, compassion, collaboration, consistency, and celebration can help reduce tension at home and arm your kids with the resources they need to realize their full potential.

Self-control

Learning and practicing self-control is crucial at any stage of life. Recognizing that raising a child with ADHD can be emotionally draining, it suggests "learning to manage your emotions initially.so that you might train your youngster to do the same."

It's probably not great for the kids when their parents internalize and ruminate on their emotional anguish. A common refrain among the children who visit her clinic is something along the lines of "If I'm dissatisfied and then you turn upset, nobody can aid me in taming it in and going to the center again. In case you decide to use it as retaliation against me, know that any loss would only add gasoline to the fire. For youngsters with ADHD, it's important to see adults who can control their emotions in challenging situations. Keep in mind that learning how to control one's emotions is a skill that can be taught to both kids and grownups through practices like mindfulness meditation.

Compassion

For someone with ADHD, each day is like being hit by a succession of "small t traumas." The cumulative effect of "a thousand paper cuts" is chipping away at these kids' healthy sense of self-worth. The first step toward helping children with ADHD understand to be kind to oneself is for people to demonstrate kindness toward them. When people constantly point out a child's shortcomings, it can damage their self-esteem. Young children often want to tell their caregivers things like, "I need you to accept and comprehend me even if I don't comprehend and appreciate myself."

51

Compassion is often defined as meeting a youngster "where they are," instead of where one thinks they should be. Parents may make a difference by loving their children no matter what and accepting them for who they are, flaws and all.

Collaboration

By maintaining their own composure and showing empathy, parents and teachers can help their charges adopt effective growth techniques. It's preferable to collaborate with kids to create solutions than to impose restrictions from on high. Typically, kids think they should have a say in matters that directly affect them. There is a constant stream of feedback from customers, and they carefully consider each suggestion. When a youngster has a stake in something, they are more likely to participate, cooperate, and gain from it.

Here's a strategy for guardians and educators: Convene and make a list of the changes you want to make to your work or school life that will make your daily routine easier. It's possible that your youngster only has two items on his or her plate, while you have fifteen. Nonetheless, you should select those two products instead, as they will likewise be on your list.

If you and your child, for instance, constantly dispute over the condition of your child's bedroom, then you and your youngster likely have a problem. Therefore, how do you go about teaching cleanliness? You are expected to take part in this activity as the adult in charge. Saying something like, "Go tidy your room," is ineffective. Before departing, they'll take a look round, find something, and exclaim, "Wow, where has this been?" An adult can serve as a "double," or a person who assists a youngster in mastering a skill, during practice sessions. Creating a shared checklist and talking through the strategy are two possible approaches to this end. Saline suggests coming up with creative ways to spice up mundane tasks. Inform them, "We're going to devote fifteen minutes and put your room together. Everyone put on some music they appreciate and we'll get started."

Consistency

Kids with ADD/ADHD do better when they have routines and structure in their day that they can count on every day. With this comes the need for standardised regulations and punishments. Always follow through on your commitments, prioritizing reliability over perfection.Children often feel betrayed by their parents when they make promises but don't follow through with

52

them. Some parents will tell their kids things like, "I'm not going to be picking up your crap anymore," and then they'll go through their kid's backpack at school and clean it up.

They won't stop pushing you since they have no idea where the limit is; this is especially frustrating for those who think in the literal sense, because as time passes, the line moves.

Celebration

Positive reinforcement is only given to children with ADHD at a rate of one-fifteenth the rate of negative reinforcement. Most kids think grown-ups care more regarding them when they "fail" than when they "succeed." A lack of positive feedback may lead to the development of feedback aversion in children and adolescents with ADHD. A child's efforts should be recognized even if they are unsuccessful.

Our goal is development through exercise, not perfection. At this stage, the process matters more than the outcome. Using this method, children can hone their executive functioning skills and become well-rounded people. The percentage of times they turned in their homework has increased from 50% to 80%. This right here is progress.

Think about the greatest way to showcase your kid's strengths. They get up and continue their daily routine of attending the same school. That's a wonderful trait to possess. Keep up that willingness to explore new things. We have done extensive research into the discrepancy. It is imperative that we put these skills to use. Kids can excel in many areas, from tech to doodling to acting; capitalize on their many interests and talents by giving them opportunities to do so.

One of the young boys I helped manage his emotions. Since he seemed open to the idea, I suggested he enroll in an improv class. As a regular at the stage for the past four years, he has found that acting has helped him with executive functioning issues including memory and focus.

Negative feedback might be difficult to reduce. If your adolescent is driving you up the wall and you can only think of one thing you're grateful for is that they're washing their hands and brushing their teeth, then this is the thing to say to them: "I can't help but notice how pleasant your scent is. Cute T-shirt.

Medication can help some kids with ADHD, but "medication don't teach skills." Children need consistent praise and instruction as they work to develop their executive functioning abilities. You should separate yourself from your sense of self. The inquiry "What's amiss with ME?" is a natural one for these teens to ask. Why do I feel so lowly? I don't understand why I keep making the same mistake. Instead, she teaches her students about how the brain works and how they can acquire greater self-control and better decision-making skills.

Putting some emotional distance between themselves and their experiences helps kids "create separation between 'what my mind is and 'what I am.'" Helping kids replace negative self-talk such as "I am a distracted person" with more positive statements such as "I am educating my mind to focus better" can have a significant impact on their ability to overcome distractions. Check out this approach I'm taking, if you please.

Using this language and providing kids with ADHD with explicit teaching in executive functioning skills is helpful. Asking kids what executive functioning abilities they will need to employ, such as changing directions from hearing to analyzing, organizing, and arranging, and offering aid if they are having problems with any of these processes, is helpful when introducing an assignment like writing a tale. Keep in mind that while talking about a child's abilities, you are talking about those abilities, not the child.

For parents whose youngsters have just been diagnosed with ADHD or who are struggling to help their children cope with daily life, some words of comfort are provided below.

The first good news is that they have a promising future. The intellect never stops developing and evolving. You can't judge your child's future by today's standards. Put an end to worrying about the future and appreciate the now.

And secondly, your efforts are not in vain."

Many kids have told me they would be lost without their parents during the day. The influence you have extends well beyond what you may think.

As a final point, she has seen many people who were initially labeled with ADHD as youngsters go on to have productive lives as adults. If a child with ADHD receives effective treatment and is given the chance to develop necessary skills, he or she can lead a fulfilling and successful life.

THE BASIC ADVICE TO HELP YOU ACCEPT AND MANAGE YOUR CHILD'S BEHAVIOR PEACEFULLY.

Parents of children and adolescents with Attention Deficit Hyperactivity Disorder (ADHD) often report feeling frustrated and worn out (ADHD or ADD). But you can help your kid take on and win over the challenges of everyday life, channel their energy in positive ways, and bring more calm to the household. As if you start making things better for your baby as early and often as you can, they will have a better chance of succeeding in life.

Children with ADHD sometimes struggle to plan ahead, stay organized, rein in their instincts, and see a project through to its conclusion. Consequently, you will have to play a more executive role in helping your child improve their executive abilities by giving them a lot of additional advise.

The youngster with attention deficit hyperactivity disorder who ignores you, frustrates you, or embarrasses you is not doing so intentionally but rather as a result of his or her hyperactivity and inattention (ADHD). Kids with ADHD want the same things as any other kid: to be obedient, to maintain their rooms, and to respect their parents' wishes.

Remembering that your kid's ADHD is equally as challenging for you may help you behave more constructively and supportively. When treated early, attention deficit hyperactivity disorder in children is manageable.

If you want to be a successful parent of a child with ADHD, you need to have a firm grasp on how your child's symptoms affect the rest of the family. When a child has attention deficit hyperactivity disorder (ADHD), they may exhibit a wide range of behaviors, many of which are disruptive at home. They "don't hear" their parents' commands, thus they routinely disobey them. Due to their lack of focus and propensity to become sidetracked, they keep the rest of the family waiting. Some people are good at starting things, but they never finish them or put in the effort to clean up after themselves. As a result of speaking before thinking, children who battle with impulsivity are more likely to say things that could be hurtful or embarrassing. Putting kids to bed and making sure they sleep through the night is not always easy. Children and teens with ADD/ADHD often act recklessly or put themselves in danger.

Many challenges arise for siblings of kids with ADHD as a result of their siblings' actions. They don't get as much help as kids who with

ADHD do. They may receive a harsher rebuke when they commit an error and less recognition when they succeed. They may be liable for the hyperactive sibling's actions and requested to help raise them. However, the affection that a sibling has for an ADHD sibling may be complicated by feelings of envy and anger on both sides.

The job of supervising an ADHD youngster might be challenging. You may experience anger, frustration, and even guilt when your child will not really "listen." Your child's behavior may be causing you stress and anxiety. If your character is significantly different from your child's, accepting their ADHD behavior may be very difficult.

Raising an ADHD child is difficult, but it can be overcome with the right balance of empathy and firmness. A home that provides both affection and stability is ideal for any young person or adolescent working to manage their attention deficit hyperactivity disorder.

Here are a few tips for becoming a more effective parent:

Stay Positive and Healthy

Care for your child's mental and physical health as your top priority if you want them to flourish as an adult. A lot of the items that can improve your child's illness signs are within your reach.

Keep your chin up and keep going. You can do a lot to help your child manage the challenges of ADHD with your positive perspective and common sense. Keeping your cool will let you connect with your child and soothe them.

It's important to keep things in perspective if you suspect your child has a mental disorder. Usually, nobody meant any harm. Maintain your humorous outlook. Perhaps in ten years from now, everyone will look back on today's most mortifying memories and find them humorous.

Do your best not to let trivial matters bother you. If your child has already performed two chores plus their homework for the day, having left one unfinished won't be a big deal. Aiming for perfection will lead to unhappiness and inappropriate expectations for your ADHD child's behavior.

Having faith in your child is important. Think about or write down all the amazing things about your child that make them unique. Have faith in your child's ability to absorb new information, adjust to change, grow, and achieve success. Consider why you can rely on this person every morning while you make coffee or clean your teeth.

As a parent, you are an inspiration to your child. You should follow suit. As a parent, it might be easy to forget of the assistance you've set up to assist your child with ADHD succeed due to exhaustion and impatience.

Seek out some aid, please. Having people believe in you and your ability to help your child is invaluable while dealing with ADHD. Communicate with your child's doctors, therapists, and teachers. Join a group that works with families who have a kid diagnosed with attention deficit hyperactivity disorder. In these communities, individuals can give and receive support while also feeling safe to open up about their own struggles and triumphs.

Soothe your weary soul with a good night's sleep. Your friends and family want to help out by offering to babysit, and while you certainly appreciate their offer, you may feel uneasy leaving your child in the hands of a complete stranger if they have attention deficit hyperactivity disorder (ADHD). If they offer to talk to you about how to manage your child again, you should consider taking them up on it.

Recuperate and take very good care of yourself. Eat well, get plenty of exercise, and find healthy ways to deal with stress like yoga or a hot bath before night. If you're sick, accept it and get help.

Establish a structure and stick to it

Regular and consistent routines in familiar settings improve children's chances of completing tasks when they have attention deficit hyperactivity disorder (ADHD). Instilling a sense of stability and self-confidence in your child is your first priority, thus it is your job to make the house a calm and safe place for everyone to live.

Helpful hints for parents of kids with ADHD:

- Maintain regularity. Creating a routine that includes a set time and location for each activity will assist the kid with ADHD better comprehend and comply with those expectations. You should establish regular times for eating, studying, playing, and sleeping. Please let your child lay out their school clothes and organize their school supplies the night before.

- Repeatedly checking the clock is a must. Have a huge clock in your child's room and other clocks around the house to serve as an example. Let your child complete tasks at his or her own pace, such as schoolwork or dressing ready for the day. Use a timer to keep track of how long it takes to complete an assignment or how long it takes to make a big transition, such when the children are calming down from playing and preparing for bed.

- Create a simple routine for your child. It's good for kids with ADHD to have things to do afterwards school, but if they have too many options, they may become distracted. The child's after-school schedule may need to be adjusted based on his or her abilities and the requirements of the activity.
- Create a tranquil setting. Let your child have some private time to unwind. The child can choose between their bedroom and the front porch for this time-out, but it should be somewhere else from the spot they normally spend their time-outs.
- Strive for order and cleanliness at all times. Put your house in order and it will feel more like a home. Instill in your child the idea that everything has a home. Put forth effort to maintain a clean and orderly workspace, and your staff will follow your lead.
- Children with ADD or ADHD may have more trouble at home if they have more time to sit around doing nothing (ADHD). A child with attention deficit hyperactivity disorder (ADHD) benefits from activity, but not too much.
- Enroll your child in lessons, whether they're art, athletics, or music. Simple yet entertaining activities will help you to keep your child occupied while you get some much-needed rest. Helping out in the household, enjoying a strategy game, or making art with a sibling are all examples of such activities. Don't spend too much time in front of the TV, at the computer, or playing video games. Your child's attention deficit hyperactivity disorder (ADHD) may be made worse by the growing violent content on TV and in computer games.

Encourage movement and sleep
Hyperactivity is a common symptom of attention deficit hyperactivity disorder in children. By taking part in competitive sports or other forms of physical activity, they can release pent-up adrenaline and learn to focus on specific activities and skills. Physical activity benefits include increased concentration, less stress, and the formation of new brain cells. However, the most important advantage of exercise for kids who have trouble paying attention is the better sleep it generally brings.

Try to find a sport that both interests and challenges your child. For youngsters who have difficulties focusing, sports like baseball that require a lot of "leisure time" are not a better match. Playing sports like basketball and hockey, which require constant movement, are ideal. Children with ADHD can benefit from both the physical and mental challenges of martial arts (such as tae kwon do) and yoga.

When kids with ADHD spend time in a park with lots of grass and trees, they show more improvement than when they spend time on a concrete playground. Keeping ADHD under control might be difficult, so remember this simple technique. Even if you live in a major city, chances are you're still close enough to a playground or other green areas to bring your kids there for some outside playtime. Gain some much-needed workout and fresh air by taking part in this "time window" with your kids.

Anyone can have trouble concentrating after not getting enough sleep, but children with ADD or ADHD may be more impacted (ADHD). Even while children with ADHD need the same level of sleep as their students without disabilities, they often don't get enough of it. One symptom of their inability to focus is that they are overstimulated and have problems sleeping. The best way to deal with this issue is to create and stick to a regular early bedtime routine.

If you want to help your child get a better night's sleep, try one or several of the following recommendations:

- You should limit your kid's TV time and encourage them to participate in other, more physical activities.
- Caffeine is not appropriate for children of any age.
- Aim for at least an hour or two of downtime before bedtime. Think about doing something like painting, reading, or playing quietly to keep oneself occupied.
- Ten minutes of close cuddling with your child. You may unwind and build a foundation of trust and affection.
- Place some fragrant lavender or other plants in your child's bedroom. There's a chance this will appeal to your child's perception of smell.

Relaxing music or a recording meditation can help your youngster go asleep. The alternatives are virtually limitless, with nature sounds and relaxing music only two examples. "White noise" can be calming for kids with ADHD. Using an electric fan or setting a radio to static will generate white noise.

Set Clear Expectations And Rules
Children with attention deficit hyperactivity disorder need consistent and simple rules they can follow. It's important to have a set of rules that everyone can follow around the house. Your kid

must be capable of comprehending the guidelines. As a result, you should commit them to paper and display them prominently.

Children with ADHD benefit greatly from well-defined systems of outcomes and rewards. It's crucial to spell out the consequences of both complying with and breaking the rules. Finally, always and consistently carry up with a form of recognition as part of your system.

While working on these consistent frameworks, keep in mind that children with ADHD are often the targets of criticism. Always keep an eye out for positive behavior and be quick to praise it. They need to be told when they've done well, especially since youngsters with ADHD are rarely praised. These kids get a lot of negative feedback and correction for their actions, but not much encouragement.

Even the smallest gestures of affection from you, such as a smile or a positive comment, can have a significant impact on your child's focus, attention span, and impulse control. Respond negatively as little as possible to improper behavior or poor work performance and instead emphasize providing positive appreciation for appropriate behavior and task completion. Don't disregard your child's smaller successes just because they aren't as big as others'.

The choice of reward and consequence is also available to you.

Rewards
- Try rewarding your youngster with special privileges, words of praise, or fun activities instead of food or toys.
- Adjust the perks on a regular basis. Kids with ADHD lose interest if they are constantly rewarded the same way.
- Make a chart that your kid may check out to see how many stars or points he or she has earned for good behavior. This will be a physical representation of all they have accomplished.
- Incremental benefits that lead up to a greater reward can be successful, but immediate incentives are more efficient than the guarantee of a future reward.

    Be sure there's a payoff for your efforts.

Consequences
- Your child's actions should be dealt with immediate and obvious consequences that you have discussed with them in advance.
- In the event of misbehavior, you may implement time-outs or the removal of perks.

- If you want to prevent your child from acting out, you need to remove them from the situations and environments that could trigger such behavior.
- If your child misbehaves, you should talk to them regarding what they might have done instead and then have them act out the better choice.
- Ensure there is always some sort of repercussion for your conduct.

Help Your Child Eat Right

Whether or not diet plays a role in the onset of ADD, it is clear that the choices you make in the kitchen have an impact on your child's mental state and, consequently, their behavior. Monitoring your child's diet in terms of what they eat, when they eat, and how much they consume, and making any required adjustments, might help alleviate symptoms of adhd disorder (ADHD).

Children do better when they eat healthy, home-cooked meals on a regular basis and avoid processed foods. The ideas presented here are applicable to children diagnosed with Attention Deficit Hyperactivity Disorder (ADHD), whose impulsivity and distraction may lead to inappropriate eating behaviors such as skipping meals, eating disorders, and obesity.

Hyperactive and impulsive kids are notorious for their erratic eating patterns. They may go without eating for a while if their parents don't intervene, and then they'll probably overeat when they finally give in. Because of this hazardous conduct, the child's physical and mental well-being may suffer.

You should not let more than three hours pass between your kid's meals and snacks, so set up a timetable that works for everyone. They won't be as likely to adopt bad eating habits as a result of this. A kid with ADHD needs to eat well on a consistent basis; mealtimes provide a mental break and a sense of routine that can help calm hyperactivity. To maintain his or her health, a youngster with ADHD should eat well on a regular basis.

- Clear up your pantry of all the processed foods you've been hoarding.

- Avoid ordering foods that are heavy in sugar and fat when eating out.

- If you don't want to see commercials promoting fast food on TV, don't watch those shows.

- A daily multivitamin and mineral supplement might be beneficial for your child.

Teach Your Child How To Make Friends
Even the most fundamental aspects of social contact can be difficult for children with ADHD. This person may misinterpret social cues, have difficulty controlling their speech, interrupt others frequently, or come across as angry or "extremely passionate." They may stand out even among youngsters of the same age because of their immature emotional development, making them easy prey for bullying.

However, keep in mind that several children with ADHD are incredibly intelligent and creative persons who, if given sufficient time, will figure out how to relate to others and detect those inappropriate acquaintances on their own. The same personality quirks that may drive their parents and teachers up the wall might be seen as humorous and endearing by their peers.

Children with ADHD have a harder time learning and adapting to new social norms and social expectations. Your child with ADHD will benefit from lessons in active listening, reading non - verbal signals, and interacting well in groups.

- Communicate with your child openly and kindly about the challenges they are facing and how they might grow.
- You should role-play different social scenarios with your child. Keep switching places and try to make it a fun time.
- Be sure your kid only plays with kids of similar intelligence and athletic prowess.
- For starters, just have a friend or two over at a time. Keep a tight eye on them and enforce a rigorous zero-tolerance policy against hitting, kicking, and screaming while they play.
- You should provide your child plenty of opportunities to play and regularly reinforce appropriate actions while they are playing.

TEACH PARENTS THAT THE CHILD IS NOT THE GUILTY

It might be difficult for parents to identify the negative patterns of behavior that are characteristic of ADHD in their children. A child's behavior may seem like simple misbehavior at first. It's normal for parents of an ADHD child to feel concerned, frustrated, or even contempt for their child.

The actions of their child may cause parents to feel embarrassed or ashamed in social situations. They may begin to wonder if their actions contributed to the problem. However, kids with ADHD have a hard time learning how to keep their focus, conduct, and energy levels steady.

Parents can better support their children in developing and achieving their potential when they have a firm grasp on ADHD and effective parenting techniques.

The challenges of raising a child with attention deficit hyperactivity disorder (ADHD) are very different from those of raising a "normal" child. You'll need to employ a number of strategies to manage the issue at home, as the nature and intensity of your child's signs can make standard rule-making and cleaning routines practically impossible. Even while some of your child's ADHD-related behaviors might become rather frustrating, there are ways to make life simpler for both you and your child.

Parents of children diagnosed with attention deficit hyperactivity disorder (ADHD) need to be aware that their baby's brains are designed differently than those of typically developing children. Children with ADHD are at an increased risk of acting impulsively, despite their ability to acquire appropriate and inappropriate behaviors.

You'll need to learn new ways of coping with your kid's ADHD symptoms and modify your own behavior if you want to aid in his or her growth. Your child's treatment plan may begin with a course of medication. Always be prepared to manage your child's ADHD symptoms with a behavioral approach. Observing these guidelines can help you raise a child who is less likely to engage in harmful conduct and more capable of overcoming self-doubt.

There are two main schools of thought within behavior management treatment that form its foundational tenets. One method is to publicly acknowledge and reward good behavior (positive reinforcement). One way to get rid of bad behavior is to make sure it never happens again is to make sure that there are consequences for it if it does happen. You may help your child learn that their behavior has consequences by establishing ground rules and providing firm punishments for infractions. These concepts should be utilized regularly throughout a child's development. The home, the classroom, and the community are all considered to be "outside" settings.

Teaching a child to modify their behavior means helping them develop the ability to consider the outcomes of potential actions and exercise self-control in the face of temptation. The parent needs empathy, patience, love, enthusiasm, and power to raise their child well. Parents should set clear limits on the kinds of behavior they'll accept from their children. Observing these norms is essential. Reprimanding a youngster for one behavior one day and ignoring it the next is counterproductive to the child's growth. Outbursts of physical abuse, unwillingness to rise from bed each morning, or disobedience when asked to turn off the tv are all behaviors that should never be permitted.

Your youngster may have difficulty comprehending and complying with your rules. Rules should be simple and easy to comprehend, and children should be awarded for following them. You can accomplish this via a points-based system. For instance, you may implement a point system where your youngster can earn rewards for good behavior, such as extra time in front of the TV or a new video game. Rules for the home should be documented and displayed where everyone can see them. Positive reinforcement and consistent repetition may help your youngster learn and follow your rules.

While it's important to consistently reward appropriate behavior and limit inappropriate ones, it's equally important not to be too strict with your child. Keep in mind that kids with ADHD could have a harder time adjusting to new environments. To help your child grow, you'll need to learn to be patient with them when they make mistakes. Strange habits that aren't causing harm to your kid or anyone else should be accepted as a natural part of your kid's character. Every person your child comes into contact with is affected by this. Attempting to modify a child's quirky behaviors simply because you think them odd is never a good idea. Perhaps it would cause more problems than it solved.

Occasionally, children with ADHD may act aggressively. The term "time-out" can be used to effectively calm down both you and your too active child. Do your best to keep your cool and remove your child from the situation if he or she acts up in public. A "time-out" should be explained to the youngster as a chance for them to collect themselves and think about why their behavior was improper. Ignoring your child's annoying habits will give them a chance to release some of their restless energy. Disruptive, abusive, or damaging behavior that goes against your rules should always be dealt with severely.

As you keep working toward embracing the child, you may find the following helpful.

Create A Workable Structure

Construct a routine for your kid, and stick to it. Establish regular times for eating, studying, playing, and sleeping. Make sure your kid has a routine, like laying out their clothes the night before so they're ready to go in the morning.

Break Tasks Into Smaller Pieces

One option is to use a large wall calendar to assist a child keep track of their obligations. Your youngster will be less likely to feel overwhelmed by their daily tasks and studies if they are assigned to different colors. Even morning tasks should be broken down into manageable chunks.

Simplify And Organize Your Life

Make sure your kid has a quiet spot where they can do their schoolwork and reading without interruption. Keep your house tidy and orderly so your kid may simply find his or her way around. It's a good way to get rid of extraneous noise and clutter.

Ensure You Have Distractions Limited

Adolescents with ADHD are more prone to prefer readily available diversions. Media like the computer, TV, and video games should be restricted since they promote impulsive behavior. Spending less time in front of tech devices and more time engaging in adventurous things outside the home will help your youngster more effectively release pent-up energy.

Encourage Exercises

Exercising is a fantastic method to burn off extra juice. Furthermore, it helps a kid focus their attention on specific tasks. You might be less rash after taking this. Positively activating the brain, improving focus, and decreasing the likelihood of experiencing mental health concerns like depression and anxiety are just a few of the many advantages of regular exercise. ADHD is quite common among elite athletes. Participating in sports may help a child with attention deficit hyperactivity disorder (ADHD) find healthy ways to channel their drive and enthusiasm.

Ensure Regulation Of Sleeping Patterns

Kids with ADHD might struggle to wind down before bedtime. When sleep is lacking, it is easier to become distracted, overly active, and careless. If you want your kid to thrive, you need to help them get enough sleep. Take away any sugary or caffeinated drinks and limit their TV time in the hours leading up to bedtime. Develop a practice for winding down at night that is both healthy and restful.

Encourage Thinking -Out Loud

Children with ADHD may find it difficult to exercise restraint. As a result, people frequently act or say without first giving it any thought. When your child is tempted to act out, it's important to get their perspective on what's going on. Knowing your child's thought process can help you guide them toward better self-control.

Believe In Your Child

Your youngster probably has no idea how much stress their condition causes. It's critical to always keep a positive and supportive demeanor. Encourage your child's positive actions by praising them when they behave nicely. Believe in your child and be hopeful despite the fact that you may be facing challenges due to ADHD.

Give Out Time For Individualized Counseling

You can't do it all. Your support and encouragement are important for your child, but they also require assistance from a trained professional. Find a therapist who can work with your child and provide them with another avenue to express themselves, such as art or music. If you require assistance, don't hesitate to get it. Many parents often neglect the mental needs of the parent since they are so preoccupied with the needs of their children. Your stress and anxiety, as well as that of your child, can be better managed with the assistance of a therapist. In addition to being a valuable outlet, parents may find local support groups to assist.

Below are also things you must not do:

You should give in to your youngster occasionally. The first two tasks you gave your child have been completed, so you may want to be more lenient with the last one. In the context of learning, even the smallest of actions can have a big impact.

Keep in mind that your child's disorder is the root cause of their behavior. Invisible to the untrained eye, attention deficit hyperactivity disorder (ADHD) is nonetheless a disability requiring special consideration. It's important to keep in mind that your child can't simply "snap out of it" or "be normal" when you find yourself getting frustrated or irritated.

Even if it seems obvious, try to keep things in perspective and take stuff one day at the time. Discomforts and embarrassments of today will seem less of a problem in the future.

Always remember that you have the last say in what is and is not acceptable behavior in your home because you are the parent. Care for and tolerate your child, but don't let him or her intimidate you or give you the impression like you can't speak up for yourself.

INNOVATIVE STRATEGIES TO MAKE LIFE WITH ADHD EASIER FOR YOUR CHILD.

When most individuals consider something like the diagnosis of ADHD (attention-deficit hyperactivity disorder), inattentiveness, impulsivity, and hyperactivity come to mind (attention-deficit hyperactivity disorder). This list of symptoms, however, does not give a full picture of the illness.

Children with attention deficit hyperactivity disorder (ADHD), sometimes known as attention deficit disorder (ADD), actually tend to exhibit a number of beneficial traits that may help them succeed in a range of contexts. Students with ADHD often show the kind of extraordinary levels of innovation, curiosity, enthusiasm, and energy seen in extremely successful businessmen and inventors.

The first and foremost step in helping children with ADHD succeed is remembering that they are individuals with their own set of challenges and abilities. Instead of seeing the unique characteristics of each person as flaws that should be concealed, we should celebrate them and utilize this as an opportunity to learn more about the people and the things they do well.

In light of this, the following strategies may be useful in supporting children with ADHD.

Give Room for Exploration of Interest

Many kids with ADHD will be curious about many things and want to learn as much as they can. Allowing them the freedom to explore these areas and gain insight into their abilities can do wonders for their sense of accomplishment and their prospects for future employment.

Embrace the Child's Strength

While kids who have ADHD may struggle to maintain attention on tasks that aren't particularly engaging, they often excel when given the opportunity to utilize their skills. Once you've identified your child's unique set of strengths, you can better support their academic endeavors in the areas that truly fascinate them. Famous investor Charles Schwab, who has ADHD and has trouble reading, says, "I was always aware of the fact that I excelled with numbers." You can also add, "I honed in on my strengths and made the most of my enthusiasm for math and economics to make a living." My weaknesses were turned into strengths.

Facilitate The Best Learning Model

Many kids with ADHD have trouble focusing, while others with the disorder tend to hyperfocus on one thing to the exclusion of everything else, making it impossible for them to move on to something else. The typical classroom environment may not be conducive to either of these behaviors. They can delve deeply into a topic without wasting time switching gears. As one teacher put it, "lost learning time is often seen when students switch subjects." The flexibility of online education makes it a great option for these kids since they can study a topic for as much as they like, moving on to something else when they become bored or staying with it if they're really into it. Children who have the ability to focus for long periods of time may find that they achieve greater success if they focus on a single subject throughout the day.

Take Frequent Breaks

Young people who have trouble focusing should take frequent breaks, whether they're at school or at home doing homework. It has been suggested that class time be broken up into thirty-minute blocks with five-minute breaks in between. It's possible that the break may re-energize the students and encourage them to finish the lesson. Having a noticeable timer that emits a sound when the rest is over is a must. One of the intervals can be spent doing something else entirely, like getting a snack or walking the dog. This strategy ensures that the kid has something fun to anticipate after the school day is over.

Create a Productive Learning Environment

Because light can be both thrilling and distracting, it's important to choose illumination that has a calming impact and create a comfortable environment for the youngster to utilize it in. You shouldn't prevent your youngster from listening to songs if it helps them concentrate. It could help to use a balance ball or a chair with tires to help with mobility. Students may benefit from holding fun yet functional objects like bouncy balls, pencils, widgets, or Velcro-fastened objects as they learn or study. They could try moving around and listening to music to see if it helps them focus better. It's been found that for some youngsters, doodling actually helps them get things done.

Online schools provide effective learning environments since children's learning environments can be tailored to their needs without distracting other students or drawing unwanted attention to themselves.

Maintain an Exercise Program

Several studies have found that physical activity improves students' academic performance, and recent studies suggest that it is especially helpful for kids with ADD/ADHD (ADHD). Associate clinical professor of psychiatry at Harvard Medical School John Ratey claims that exercise can boost focus and mood just as effectively as medicine. The so-called executive processes of ordering, working memory, sorting, suppressing, and maintaining attention are activated by physical exertion, as he explains. Additionally, it helps kids be more open-minded and less prone to making hasty decisions.

Once you and your kid have learned to deal with the signs of ADHD which might interfere with learning, it's important to take a step back and consider the benefits of the disorder and act as an advocate for your child. One positive aspect of having a child with ADHD is that they are more likely to think outside the box. For kids with ADHD, an online education can be a lifesaver because of the individualized approach taken by most teachers.

Provide Positive Attention

It's not easy being a caregiver to a kid who has attention deficit hyperactivity disorder. When dealing with children, even the most tolerant of parents might run out of steam and words to say. However, investing time and energy into a youngster who has ADHD that way is well worth it.

Having fun and playing constructive games can help reduce attention-seeking actions. Also, the results will be more powerful as a result. No matter how difficult your child is to be around, you should spend time alone with them every day. One of the quickest and most successful ways to deal with behavioral issues is to give a child compliments, even if just for 15 minutes.

Give Effective Instructions

Children who struggle to pay attention need extra help when it comes to carrying out instructions. In many cases, they simply don't pay attention at the very start and miss the initial instructions. If you want your child to learn as much as possible from your instructions, the first step is to get your youngster's complete attention. Turn off the TV, make eye contact, and tap your child on the shoulder before asking for them.

Never give a series of orders such, "Have your shoes on, clean your bedroom, and then bring out the garbage." A youngster with ADHD might put on their socks before heading to their room, but once there, they could look for something else to do rather than tidy up. Each step must be explained separately.

Don't just tell someone to "clean their room" and expect them to do it. Instead of doing this, offer a good checklist or assign individual tasks, like making the bed, sorting the laundry, putting away the books, etc. Asking your child to repeat what they heard is a good way to gauge their level of comprehension.

Praise Your Child's Effort

Acknowledge your child's good deeds and tell them how proud you are of them. Providing children with ADHD with frequent feedback and positive reinforcement can help them improve their behavior.

Take care to be specific in your compliments to others. Don't just say, "Nice job;" be more precise by saying, "Great job putting your plate in the dishwasher right when I asked you to." Praising your child for good behavior, such as sitting still, following directions, and playing quietly, may help them continue this pattern.

Make Use of Time-Out When Necessary

Children with ADHD may benefit from a time-out as a way to relax their bodies and minds. A time-out can be used as a mild form of discipline as well. It's more of a fantastic life ability that can be useful in many contexts.

Teach your youngster to go to a calm, quiet location when they feel overwhelmed. Create a relaxing environment and guide them there gently, not as a form of punishment but to help them unwind. Don't fret; your child will discover out how to reach their destination before getting into difficulties on their own.

Ignore Mild Misbehaviors

Children with attention deficit hyperactivity disorder often engage in actions that are aimed at getting others to notice them. Paying attention to them in any way, even negatively, will only encourage them to keep doing what they're doing.

Ignoring them when they act up will teach them that being disruptive won't get them what they want. Don't pay attention to the whining, complaining, loud noises, or other interruptions that may be made. Eventually, your kid will put a stop to it.

Give Room for Natural Consequences

When attempting to reprimand a child who has attention deficit hyperactivity disorder, pick your battles carefully. You don't want your kid to think they're a bad person who can't get out of trouble or accomplish anything. Both of you can benefit from lowering your standards for some behaviors.

Rather of trying to persuade a youngster to make a more appropriate choice, it may be more helpful to just let the child face the results of his or her behavior. For example, if your child refuses to stop playing in order to eat lunch, you may need to remove all food from the bedroom.

As a result, it's only natural that youngsters will get hungry before dinner, and they'll have to learn to wait it out. They will be more eager to eat tomorrow's lunch because of the anticipation of the novelty.

Create A Reward System

Reward systems can be quite helpful in helping children with ADHD maintain their focus and attention. Traditional incentive systems work well for most kids, but they can be boring for kids with ADHD because they make them wait too long for a reward. If you're looking for a way to motivate your child to do the little things that add up over time, consider making a replacement behavior for them.

Choose a few desired behaviors, such as sitting at the dinner table while eating, petting a pet softly, or stashing toys after play, that will be rewarded with tokens. The next stage is to allow users to exchange tokens for more valuable rewards, like extended playtime on electronic gadgets or a chance to take part in a game the whole family enjoys.

Work Hand-In-Hand with Your Child's Teacher

Working together, parents and teachers can greatly improve a student's chances of thriving in the classroom. In order for some students to succeed in class, it may be necessary to modify their required tasks, such as providing them with additional time on tests.

Possible behavioral adjustments are also called for. Kids with ADHD may have a harder time maintaining self-control if they are forced to remain indoors during recess. As a result, you and your child should work together to create a behavior management strategy that will help them deal with their symptoms.

Having a behavior control strategy that can be used in both the home and at school can be helpful. A youngster could, for example, earn tokens or points at school and then exchange them for rewards at home.

A DEEPER LOOK AT ADHD AND HOW IT AFFECTS THE BRAIN

Adults, children, and the elderly are all susceptible to developing symptoms of ADHD. It is believed that the disease stems from a hypersensitive tendency to environmental stimulation and a failure to efficiently discriminate between irrelevant and crucial stimuli, both of which are required to complete tasks and interact with others in a meaningful and productive manner. The effects of this faulty filtering system can typically be reduced to four aspects of mental ability:

- Selective attention allows us to focus on what we need to in order to get our jobs done. When the brain is unable to filter irrelevant information and focus on what's most important, the result can be bad selective attention, which manifests itself in a variety of ways, including a failure to pay close enough attention to details, the making of careless mistakes, the propensity to be caught off guard and forgetful, the misplacing of objects, and the inability to pay attention to what other people are saying.
- When we pay attention over long periods of time, we are better able to solve problems and move forward. Some people are easily distracted, making it challenging for them to accomplish prolonged or hard tasks, or even to read for long periods of time, without getting bored.
- Controlling our impulses enables us to assess the appropriateness of our responses and the appropriateness of those responses. Interrupting others, speaking too quickly, and jumping to conclusions without considering all the facts are just a few of the issues that can arise when one is impulsive.
- Being in control of our impulses allows us to gauge the appropriateness of our responses and the timeframe of those responses. Interrupting others, speaking too quickly, and making hasty decisions without collecting and processing all of the information needed to do so are just a few of the ways in which impulsivity can cause trouble.
  In most cases, attention deficits become apparent when they interfere with a person's ability to perform important daily tasks like cleaning, cooking, or attending to schoolwork. Some of the symptoms include;
- Problems with organization can lead to a feeling of disarray and make it harder to keep things under control.

- Being readily sidetracked by irrelevant information or irrelevant ideas, to the point where careless errors are made frequently while performing tasks.
- daydreaming or thinking otherwise when being addressed by others (e.g., a teacher, employee, or loved one).
- In a forgetful mood.
- Problems staying focused for extended periods of time while doing things like reading or viewing a film.
- Having a strong aversion to doing things for extended periods of time that need one to maintain focus and pay close attention, such as writing a lengthy paper or a reference, counting inventory, paying taxes, or folding and packing up laundry.
- Since I am easily sidetracked, I am having a hard time getting my work done on time.
- Basic day-to-day functioning and relationship quality can be considerably affected when both unresponsive and hyperactivity-impulsivity signs are present. Problems with hyperactivity and impulsivity aren't always tied to attention deficits, but it's not uncommon for both to coexist.

Below is a review from a person living with ADHD:
A diagnosis of one form of ADHD does not guarantee that a person will always display the symptoms typical of that form or that they will always be able to be neatly classified as having ADHD. There will be days when people are more hyperactive than usual, days when they are more inattentive than usual, and days when they are both. In the talks, the most typical consequences of possessing ADHD are discussed. While I tend to be unfocused, I have days where I can't seem to shut up, am constantly fidgeting (a hallmark of adult hyperactivity), or have a hard time reining in my impulses. Our primary appearance might also change over time, especially as we mature and learn more about ourselves. ``
ADHD can be difficult to detect externally, especially in older people. To live normally in a culture that was not designed to suit our unique brains and that is not necessarily particularly comprehending the difficulties or demands we confront, those of us with ADHD learn to hide our symptoms and keep our problems to ourselves. We also develop strategies for dealing with everyday challenges that help us function more effectively and make our ADHD less noticeable to the outside world.

Most people wrongly assume that the primary symptom of ADHD is a general lack of focus. This is owed in part to the myths surrounding ADHD, but also to the nomenclature of the condition. Attention Deficit Hyperactivity Disorder is the proper label for this ailment. The illness is sometimes misunderstood as a failure to pay attention when, in fact, it is characterized by problems with self-control. Our inability to regulate our energy levels, focus, emotions, actions, and impulses is a direct result of individual differences in brain structure and function.

To sum up, the issue is not the fact that we lack the ability to focus; rather, it is that we have difficulty focusing our attention where it needs to be and on the right things. If you're trying to focus on something unappealing, like paying bills or listening to a lecture, you're bound to get distracted by something more interesting. A mind unaffected by attention deficit hyperactivity disorder is able to take a breath, determine that a particular stimulus is irrelevant, choose to dismiss it, and then resume to the task at hand.

People with ADHD have a harder time suppressing their reaction to a distraction, so they are more likely to devote it some of their focus. Then, because of working memory issues, we may find it difficult to get back on track with what we were doing before we were distracted. Because of the challenges we face in regulating our attention, there are times when we work to offer the optimal amount of attention and other instances when we strive to give too much.

How ADHD Affects the Brain

Individuals who suffer from Attention Deficit Hyperactivity Disorder (ADHD) differ from individuals who do not suffer from the disorder in terms of how their brains developed, how they are structured, and how they perform. These differences are critical for understanding and treating some ADHD-related behaviors and symptoms.

In comparison to people who do not suffer from ADHD, those with the disorder show different neurological differences. Variations due to Attention Deficit Hyperactivity Disorder are evident in

- brain structure
- functions of the brain
- brain development

Brain volume, neurotransmitters, and neural circuitry are all linked to these morphological shifts. It's probable that those with ADHD experience delayed or altered brain maturation compared to those without the disorder. As a kid grows up, his or her brain could change in unexpected ways.

The method through which the baby's mind develops varies with the child's developmental age. These steps, identified in an earlier study from a reputable source, include:

- Neurons are the brain's cellular units of communication, and they need to be carefully nurtured, placed, and organized into functional brain networks.
- Because myelin sheaths protect and insulate neurons, nerve impulses can travel more efficiently from one cell to another.
- Neurite pruning involves the rewiring of brain regions when activity is thought to be inefficient or unnecessary.

ADHD can have a wide range of effects on brain function. Cognitive, behavioral, and motivational problems have been linked to this illness. Hyperactivity-hyperactivity disorder (ADHD) can disrupt both the brain's ability to regulate emotions and its ability to form new connections between neurons. As a corollary, it may cause a breakdown in coordination between the various regions of the brain.

Neurons, the brain's nerve cells, are clustered together to transmit signals to different parts of the brain. It has been hypothesized that individuals with attention deficit hyperactivity disorder (ADHD) have brain networks that develop more slowly and are less effective at transferring specific messages, behaviors, or information. It's possible that separate sections of these brain networks are responsible for distinct activities including attention, movement, and emotion.

Brains of people with neurodevelopmental disorders like ADHD can be imaged using MRIs and X-rays to detect subtle differences in brain structure and function. Inattentional and hyperactivity disorder (ADHD) are examples of such conditions. Imaging studies of people with ADHD have revealed a disproportion in the development of certain brain networks, a phenomenon known as structural connectivity. The dysfunctional connectivity between some brain networks is another issue.

Scientists and doctors can see how persons with ADHD's brains differ from those of neurotypical people by comparing the activity pattern across different brain areas. These experiments aim to provoke a certain mental state by, for example, posing difficult questions or eliciting strong feelings.

Recent studies have shown that people with ADHD have "hyperactive" and "hypoactive" brain regions. This suggests that the brain's computing complexity may not be sufficient to meet the mental effort of the activity.

A person with attention deficit hyperactivity disorder (ADHD) may, for example, have trouble turning down the volume on their brain's default attention network. When the difficulty level of the task at hand rises, this becomes even more apparent. There may be a correlation between this and an increased inclination for distraction.

The following are some of the areas of executive functioning that ADHD can impact:

Abilities in paying attention, focusing, concentrating, remembering, remembering details, being impulsive, being hyperactive, being organized, having friends, being motivated, making decisions, switching tasks, and learning from mistakes.

Both those with and without ADHD have distinctively different brain structures. These alterations have a wide-ranging impact on many brain regions associated with classic ADHD symptoms.

Many children with attention deficit hyperactivity disorder (ADHD) have delayed brain development and/or have smaller brain volumes than typically developing children. The amygdala and the hippocampus, which are involved in controlling emotions, memory, and motivation, are only two regions of the brain that frequently show volume differences. It's crucial to keep in mind that a larger brain size has no correlation to higher intelligence.

Some regions of the brain of children with ADHD develop more slowly than others. The frontal lobes, which are responsible for cognitive control, focus management, and planning control, showed the most significant lags. ADHD symptoms, such as agitation and fidgeting, may be related to the motor cortex maturing faster than average in children with ADHD.

The frontal lobe regulates a wide range of mental operations, such as focus, impulse management, and appropriate social behavior. Adults with attention deficit hyperactivity disorder may develop more slowly than average in certain areas of the prefrontal cortex. Delaying treatment could cause permanent damage to these cognitive processes.

The frontal lobe's premotor cortex and prefrontal cortex regulate motor activity and attention, respectively. There is some evidence that people with ADHD have reduced brain activity in specific regions.

Inattention ADHD is a neurodevelopmental condition that causes changes in brain size, shape, and function. Delays in development and abnormalities in the functioning of numerous regions of the brain are also associated with attention deficit hyperactivity disorder (ADHD). Individual differences in the ADHD brain can have far-reaching effects on how these individuals think, act, and feel.

The lack of norepinephrine was considered to be the cause of ADHD, making it the first disorder to be linked to a specific neurotransmitter deficit. Medication created specifically to address this physiologic deficit was first successfully applied to the treatment of ADHD. Norepinephrine, like all the other neurotransmitters, is made in the brain. All norepinephrine molecules have dopa as their primary building block. This little molecule gets converted into dopamine, which subsequently gets converted into norepinephrine.

Abnormal neurotransmitter activity has been linked to hyperactivity-hyperactivity disorder in four brain areas:

- **Frontal cortex**: This part of the brain coordinates complex mental processes, such as paying attention and staying organized. Issues with focus, disorganization, and executive function may result from a shortage of norepinephrine in this brain region.
- **Limbic system**: A more inwardly located region of the brain regulates our emotional state. Irritability, distractedness, and emotional vulnerability are all symptoms of a deficit in this area.
- **Basal ganglia**: The communication mechanisms in the brain are managed by these neural circuits. The basal ganglia act as a relay station, collecting data from across the brain and relaying it to where it needs to go. A deficiency in the basal ganglia can cause a "short-circuiting" of information, which manifests as inattention or impulsive conduct.
- **Reticular activating system**: From the many pathways that enter and leave the brain, this is probably the most crucial relay system. It's possible that problems in the RAS underlie attentional difficulties, impulsivity, and hyperactivity.

ADHD is a commonly diagnosed disease in children who show these brain changes in addition to the conventional symptoms. The condition can be managed, and in some cases the symptoms lessen with time. Many patients report increased happiness and success in school after receiving therapy for their ADHD.

HOW TO MAKE SURE YOU GET THE RIGHT DIAGNOSIS

Even though ADD/ADHD is frequently diagnosed, that does not mean it should be diagnosed carelessly. Other "resources" are not backed by research and aren't worth your effort and money because they are not part of a standard examination of ADHD that includes multiple conventional and complex diagnostic techniques. Sorting out which is which is the real test.

In order to diagnose attention deficit hyperactivity disorder, a qualified medical professional must do a thorough physical examination (ADHD). An accurate and complete diagnosis of ADHD requires a clinical assessment, a review of the patient's condition, and the execution of normed assessment scale by the child's dear ones, educators, and colleagues. It's a lengthy procedure with several stages.

ADHD can only be properly diagnosed by a medical professional. A child psychiatrist, a psychiatric nurse practitioner, or even an APRN might be the right fit here (APRN). But keep in mind that just because someone has a certain accreditation doesn't mean they are expert at spotting ADHD and its co-occurring disorders. While the most qualified medical and nursing professionals routinely seek out more training, the vast majority have never gotten enough instruction in diagnosing and evaluating ADHD. Ask your doctor how experienced they are with identifying ADHD and how familiar they are with treating common co-occurring disorders. To be successful in this demanding field, one needs not a certificate but rather extensive training.

Multiple factors must be considered in order to provide a comprehensive and holistic evaluation of ADHD, such as:

- **DSMD -V for ADHD diagnosis:** To determine whether or not a patient has attention deficit hyperactivity disorder (ADHD), a doctor will first conduct a physical examination. At least six symptoms of inattention, hyperactivity, or impulsivity must have been present in patients before the age of 12. Despite its continued use as a diagnostic standard, the DSM-V has been criticized by many experts, including me, for failing to adequately address issues related to children's emotional regulation and executive functioning. When making a diagnosis, most doctors go beyond the DSM-V and do in-depth clinical interviews.

- **Clinical diagnosis for ADHD diagnosis**: The best way to determine if a person has attention deficit hyperactivity disorder is for a medical or mental health clinician familiar with ADHD and the other medical or mental health disorders that produce similar symptoms to conduct a thorough interview with the individual in question. (and, if feasible, with one or two other individuals who are aware that person well) (ADHD). It is important to ask questions like these during the clinical interview.
  - The problems that prompted the review request in the first instance
  - Daily performance at the patient's overall school of study or work, as well as in the patient's family and social relationships, based on the patient and those closest to the patient,
  - Exciting activities that a person enjoys doing for her own sake.
  - How the sufferer sees himself in the eyes of others
  - Location of Present Dwelling
  - Descended from an established ancestry Recent years have been stressful due to family strain or other factors.
  - Brain scans reveal family's emotional past
  - Nutritional and sleep patterns, as well as the development of one's body and mind.
  - Suggested expressions of emotion

  This part of the evaluation is vastly more involved than the inquiry "Why do you think your child may have ADHD?" suggests.

  If a patient reports, "I have difficulties focusing," the doctor should question, "When are you having trouble focusing?" What triggers your awareness of it? How soon before we start to see the effects of this problem? If it's the former, how long have you been noticing this trend? Mood problems and learning challenges, for instance, might cause sudden and unexplained changes in one's ability to focus and concentrate.

  The doctor should be on the lookout for patterns that could point to ADHD as the underlying cause of the diagnosis, but should also consider other possibilities. Diagnosing attention deficit hyperactivity disorder (ADHD) is not a "all or nothing" scenario; exhibiting particular symptoms does not entail a diagnosis; what does merit a prognosis are continuous and unpleasant symptoms that develop over time in two or more settings. When deciding whether or not to treat a patient, doctors must consider whether or not their symptoms are interfering with the patient's daily life.

The patient's most important sources of discomfort and the circumstances adding to its expression at work, education, or close connections can be better understood by the doctor after a thorough clinical interview. It must contain the following elements:

- Problems, signs
- Possession of strengths and abilities
- The stresses of daily living and the obligations of family life.
- For kids: just how they are doing in school as assessed by things like their test scores and grades, how lengthy it takes kids to complete tests, if they they can complete homework without parental help, and so on.
- Meeting deadlines, being efficient, etc., are all examples of how well an adult performs at work.
- The state of the patient's health in general, including their eating and sleeping habits
- , the patient's family's medical history, including any known cases of ADHD
- Use of both legal and illegal drugs
- "Previous assessments, if any, and the results of previous evaluations"
- Comorbid issues, such as depression, anxiety, and learning disabilities, are common among those with ADHD.

However, this is a deviation from the norm that very young children should not take part in clinical interviews since they often cannot correctly articulate how they are behaving or acting. Most kids can give reliable answers to clinical questions, and it's important to ask their parents, too (ideally until they're in college). Adult patients have the choice to bring a partner or trusted friend to their appointments to shed further light on their symptoms and difficulties.

In the course of a two- or three-hour clinical interview, you must spend some time going over the current understanding of ADHD and what that means for the individual patient. Not everyone has the luxury of spending an hour or more with each client; pediatricians, for example, typically have only fifteen minutes to spend with each child. In such cases, it may be necessary to have the patient come back for a second or third appointment before a sufficient amount of information is delivered.

- **Normed rated scale for ADHD diagnosis:**
  Self-report information from the patient and observer data from parents, teachers, partners, or other people who have seen this person function over recent months and previously in different aspects of daily life should be gathered using normed ADHD rating scales like the Barkley, BASC, Brown, Conners, or BRIEF scales, in addition to the clinical interview. Psychoeducational testing, which incorporates tests of intelligence as well as assessments of academic performance, might be useful if a learning disability is suspected.
- The doctor should first find out how much the patient and their loved ones know about ADHD before providing a clear and comprehensive description of the disorder. After completing each section, the doctor should pause and consult with the patient to assess the accuracy with which each section has been reported during the preceding six months.
- The doctor should reassure the patient that all of the ADHD symptoms are normal human difficulties when discussing a possible diagnosis. Many people mistakenly believe that ADHD is a binary diagnosis like pregnancy, but in reality, it has a wide range of symptoms. It's more in line with depression (everyone gets down sometimes), but we don't call someone clinically depressed unless their symptoms cause significant impairments in their day-to-day performance for a considerable amount of time.
- **Physical exam for ADHD diagnosis**:
  Sometimes, conditions within the body, including thyroid problems or pinworms, can cause symptoms that are similar to those associated with attention deficit hyperactivity disorder (ADHD). A thorough physical examination by a family doctor or pediatrician will help alleviate any fears that a health problem has been overlooked. A person's physical health is another factor that can be considered while deciding whether or not to provide ADHD medication.
- **Learning disability considerations in an ADHD diagnosis**:
  Most kids with attention deficit hyperactivity disorder also have trouble in school. As well as sharing commonalities at the genetic level, ADHD and learning disabilities also share commonalities in terms of overlapping cognitive processes, such as working memory. Several standardized exams are available for use by schools to determine whether or not students' reading, writing, and/or mathematics instruction needs to be modified.

- ○ Woodcock-Johnson Cognitive Abilities Put to the Test
- ○ Individual Achievement Test Developed by Wechsler (WIAT)
- ○ The Wechsler Intelligence Scale for Children, the Nelson-Denny Reading Test, and the (WISC-V)
- **Knowledge gauge for ADHD diagnosis**: The doctor should first find out what the patient and their loved ones already know about ADHD before providing a clear and comprehensive description of the disorder. After completing each section, the doctor should pause and consult with the patient to assess the accuracy with which each section has been reported during the preceding six months.
  - ○ A doctor discussing a possible diagnosis with a patient should stress that all of ADHD's symptoms are problems that everyone faces occasionally. Many people mistakenly believe that ADHD is a binary diagnosis like pregnancy, but in reality, it has a wide range of symptoms. It's more in line with depression (everyone gets down sometimes), but we don't call someone clinically depressed unless their symptoms cause significant impairments in their day-to-day performance for a considerable amount of time.
  - ○ The doctor should stress to the individual that assessing ADHD is an ongoing procedure. In circumstances where medicine was prescribed, it is very important to schedule a follow-up appointment with the comprehensive care to gauge the treatment's success. It is the doctor's responsibility to monitor for side effects and assess the efficacy of the current medication regimen in meeting the patient's needs at all times of.
  - ○ Let's say a person takes a medicine and finds out it has unwanted side effects or doesn't help them the way they hoped it would. They need to be encouraged to talk to their doctor about it in that scenario. Adjusting a person's medication significantly to find the best dose for them is often necessary.

What Does Not Help With ADHD Diagnosis
Despite their popularity, the following methods of diagnosis are not accepted by all doctors. In any case, you might be familiar with at least one of these testing gadgets. The following are not reliable in my experience as ADHD diagnostic tools:
- **Spect Brain imaging for ADHD diagnosis:** SPECT brain imaging makes use of radioactive processes to record blood flow in specific areas of the brain in three dimensions over the course of several minutes. As far as the individual is concerned, it is completely painless. SPECT imaging is not particularly useful for diagnosing

ADHD because it only provides information on brain activity during the brief time the test is being given. However, it is useful for evaluating specific types of brain or organ functioning after injury or disease. In determining if or not an individual has attention deficit hyperactivity disorder (ADHD), nevertheless, it is not particularly useful. It doesn't show how the mind works in other settings, like school, home life, or social interactions.

- **Computer games for ADHD diagnosis**: The player in a computer game needs to have lightning-fast reactions to specified signals flashing on the screen while ignoring other signals flashing on the screen that serve as decoys. These games, which are often boring, test and score the player on how well they can reply quickly and precisely to some indications on the computer while trying to ignore other signals. The computer will be able to compare your test results with those of other individuals who took the same tests, but it won't be able to tell you how attentive and responsive you'll be in situations where there are more complex stimuli and responses required, like in college classes, reading, or conversing with others.

- **Genetics Testing for ADHD diagnosis**: Some companies are profiting on the growing interest in the genetics of ADHD by providing so-called "genetic tests." After patients mail in a saliva or blood sample, they receive an overview of their genetics. The patient's susceptibility to numerous diseases may be outlined in this synopsis. Tests like this only look at a few of genes, although many more than that are likely involved in ADHD's hereditary make-up. No genetic test has yet been developed that can reliably predict whether or not an individual suffers from attention deficit hyperactivity disorder (ADHD).

- **Neuropsychological Testing for ADHD diagnosis**: A neuropsychologist will ask you a battery of questions and give you puzzles to solve over the course of two to four hours as part of an evaluation. Individuals are evaluated on their ability to recall a variety of words, phrases, numbers, or designs; correctly identify the colors or sayings on a set of flashcards presented in a prescribed order; and sequentially place small pegs into a pegboard using just one hand. The outcomes of these exams can be used to diagnose dementia and assess the extent of brain damage after a head trauma or stroke.

Unfortunately, these procedures cannot foretell how a healthy individual would respond to everyday situations and tasks.

The key problem with these three sorts of testing is that they aim to determine how effectively a person's brain performs in very limited and particular scenarios. Neither the intricacy nor the frequency of these scenarios is comparable to the real-world contexts in which adults must perform.

An damage to the brain is ruled out as a potential trigger for attention deficit hyperactivity disorder. It's a problem that makes it hard to focus, concentrate, and finish things, among other things, because it affects multiple brain functions and the person's intrinsic motivations. The brain's anatomy is completely normal. It affects the way a child's executive functions work in different situations.

This is what I mean when I say that the "central mystery of ADHD" is that almost all people with ADHD can exercise their executive functions very well for definite tasks or situations that are fascinating to them or when they believe that something they do not want to happen is going to occur if they do not accomplish some specific action or behavior immediately. The fact that practically everyone with ADHD is able to effectively use their executive functions is often cited as the "central riddle of ADHD." An illustration of this could be the marketing specialist who can focus very well when playing games or making a meal at home but fails to focus when working on their obligations at work. It begs the question, "Why are you able to do it in this one situation but not in others?" if this is indeed the case. It's sometimes assumed incorrectly that this is due to weak willpower, but that's not the case. A deficiency in the brain's electrochemical signaling of its self-management system is the true cause of attention deficit hyperactivity disorder (ADHD).

Negative effects on work and school performance, interpersonal connections, and overall quality of life have been associated with untreated attention deficit hyperactivity disorder (ADHD).

The following are some of the risks adults face if they have untreated ADHD:

- Adults with attention deficit hyperactivity disorder tend to be pessimistic because of the challenges the disorder presents to daily life. Low self-esteem is a common result of these problems. Adult ADHD has been linked to decreased levels of self-esteem, according to studies, although this is treatable and can be improved with therapy.

85

- Fifty percent of those who have ADHD also deal with anxiety. Medication and talk therapy are effective treatments including both attention deficit hyperactivity disorder (ADHD) and anxiety.
- Research has revealed that people with ADHD often struggle to control their emotions, which can cause problems in interpersonal relationships (poor ability to manage emotions). Irrational feelings like irritation, impatience, and anger can be hard to manage when ADHD isn't treated. When people conduct negatively in response to their emotions, it can strain relationships. Medication and therapy to enhance social and communication abilities can help those with ADHD.

- Adults with attention deficit hyperactivity disorder (ADHD) experience a number of difficulties at work including a lack of social skills, the ability to focus on a task without being interrupted, and the ability to manage complex tasks. It's possible that issues like these could lead to a lack of job security. Participating in psychotherapy can help one acquire the skills essential for managing ADHD in a professional setting. It is also important to choose a career that makes use of the abilities of ADHD, such as those found in fast-paced environments.

- When compared to the general population, people with ADHD are three times more likely to develop a nicotine addiction, as shown by the results of multiple research. Compared to those without ADHD, people with ADHD were at a 50% greater risk of developing a drug or alcohol use disorder. Research shows that drug misuse decreases when ADHD is treated with medication.

- Unintentional injury and suicide are the leading causes of death among adults with ADHD, as documented by several research. However, long-term treatment with ADHD medications substantially lowers the danger of both accidental injury and suicide.

However, it is generally possible to diagnose ADHD by monitoring a person's actions and assessing if they are consistent with the actions and behaviors of people who have been diagnosed with ADHD. Some people with ADHD may be difficult to diagnose because they suppress or mask their symptoms in order to look neurotypical.

While this may benefit individuals in the short-term with things like employment, schoolwork, and social interactions, the energy expended and the stress incurred by these measures can be detrimental to their health in the long-term.

The signs of ADHD might be hidden in those who have it, leading to a multiplicity of diagnoses and other health problems. According to the NIH, almost eight out of ten adults with ADHD also suffer from another condition, while the CDC reports that roughly six out of every 10 children with ADHD also have another diagnosis.

Specifically when other mental illnesses are included, the manifestations of ADHD in different people might differ substantially.

Any of the following conditions may be misdiagnosed as ADHD in a given patient. The presence of ADHD does not rule out the possibility of having any of these other diseases, as they can all coexist with ADHD.

Depressive Disorders

People with ADHD often have difficulty with memory, initiating tasks, and maintaining focus. It's possible that these issues with your ability to make important decisions are indicators of depression. Further, people with ADHD often battle with low self-esteem due to the frustration and uncertainty they experience as a result of their problems and the messages they receive from others claiming they are "lazy" or "just not actually trying enough."

Someone who has problems focusing due to depression may find that their concentration improves when they are not going through a depressive episode. Medications for depression may help alleviate symptoms if your condition is primarily characterized by sadness. Depression as well as other mental health conditions are caused by chemical imbalances in the brain, making it difficult to notice the symptoms.

Anxiety

ADHD and anxiety share symptoms such as restlessness, difficulty sitting still, easily becoming overwhelmed, and a lack of focus. Many people with ADD/ADHD also suffer from anxiety as a coping technique (ADHD). Increasing cortisol and adrenaline levels may help people with ADHD concentrate in the short term, but they have no lasting positive effects.

If you have problems focusing due of worry, you may find that your concentration improves as your symptoms of anxiety lessen. However, if your anxiety is decreasing while you're having more trouble focusing, your ADHD may be hiding under the surface.

If anxiety is the underlying reason of your inability to focus, you'll feel more anxious before you have trouble focusing. If you notice that your anxiety levels grow whenever you experience concentration difficulties, it's possible that the attention difficulty is actually what's causing your anxiety.

Oppositional defiant disorder

The most noticeable symptom of oppositional defiant disorder (ODD), a disease of impulse control, is disruptive behavior. Oppositional defiant disorder is characterized by persistent problems such as dishonesty, task rejection, irritability, and frequent conflicts with peers and authority figures.

In most cases, ODD presents itself in infancy, however it can also emerge during adolescence.

As a result of their hyperactivity, children with ADHD can occasionally act out in unfriendly or difficult ways. ODD, on the other hand, is not something a person is born with and can occur as a result of being ignored or abused, contrasting ADHD, which is a variance in brain function that remains throughout a person's life. Furthermore, if given the right care and encouragement, children with ODD can sometimes grow out of it. Although ADHD can be managed and its symptoms regulated, an individual who has successfully managed their symptoms is nonetheless diagnosed as having ADHD.

Bipolar disorder

Even though ADHD is a condition that people are born with, the symptoms may not always be present in childhood. Many people can thrive through high school because of the structure that was provided by the school system as well as the supervision that their parents or guardians provided. The first time that people realize they are struggling is when they enter college. Due to scheduling flexibility and diminished oversight, attention problems and impulsive behaviors can surface.

This can sometimes give the impression that the symptoms result from a new mental health problem rather than a preexisting neurodivergence that was not previously created any behaviors or functional concerns. However, this is not always the case. There is a possibility of confusing these symptoms with the manic or hypomanic phases of bipolar disorder.

"Racing thoughts" are a common symptom of attention deficit hyperactivity disorder (ADHD), which describes the sensation that one's thoughts are moving quickly and switching topics frequently. They may also have trouble falling asleep because their thoughts continue to run through their head once they lie down. In addition, although people with ADHD are said to have attended "deficits," they frequently have the ability to hyperfocus on things that are of interest to them.

Sometimes, episodes of mania or hypomania are misdiagnosed as being caused by these cognitive patterns and actions. You may have attention deficit hyperactivity disorder (ADHD) if your hyperactive symptoms are continuing or persistent. The duration of hypomanic and manic symptoms often ranges from a few weeks to a few months before they begin to improve. When attempting to differentiate between ADHD and bipolar disorder, providers need to ascertain whether symptoms are persistent or episodic and when symptoms first appeared.

MANAGING LONG-TERM SYMPTOMS WITH MEDICAL AND NONMEDICAL INTERVENTIONS

When a child is diagnosed with attention-deficit/hyperactivity disorder (ADHD), their parents frequently have concerns regarding the treatment that should be administered. With the appropriate treatment, ADHD can be brought under control. There are various treatments, and the most effective one may vary from child to child and family to family. Parents must work closely with others involved in their kid's life, such as healthcare providers, therapists, teachers, coaches, and other family members, to identify the best possibilities for their child.

Many different approaches can be taken to treat ADHD, including Medications and behavior treatment, which may also include training for the parents.

Before turning to medication as a treatment option for children with ADHD under six years old, the American Academy of Pediatrics (AAP) suggests that parents first receive training in managing their children's behaviors. The suggestions include medication and behavior treatment for children aged 6 and older; parent training in behavior management is recommended for children aged 6 to 12, and various types of behavior therapy and training are recommended for teenagers. Additionally, schools may be incorporated into the therapeutic plan. The AAP also recommends including behavioral classroom intervention and school support in the list of suggestions.

Not only can attention deficit hyperactivity disorder (ADHD) damage a child's ability to pay attention or sit still in school, but it also affects their interactions with their family and other children. Children with ADHD frequently exhibit behaviors that can be quite upsetting to those around them. It is typically important to begin behavior therapy as soon as a diagnosis is made since it is a treatment option that can help reduce these behaviors; behavior therapy is an option that can help reduce these behaviors.

The primary objectives of behavior therapy are to acquire or improve desirable patterns of conduct and to reduce or eliminate undesirable or problematic patterns of behavior. Some components of behavior treatment for ADHD include

Training for parents in managing challenging behaviors, behavior therapy with children, and behavioral interventions in the school are all options.

These methods can also be combined to achieve the desired results. When it comes to helping children enrolled in early childhood programs, it is typically most beneficial for parents and educators to collaborate on assisting the kid.

Parent Training In Behavior Management for ADHD

A child's conduct, self-control, and self-esteem can all significantly improve via behavior therapy, which is an effective treatment for attention deficit/hyperactivity disorder (ADHD). When administered by parents, it is the most successful in treating young children. Behavior therapy is something that healthcare providers should propose to the parents of children who are younger than 12 years old, according to the recommendations of experts. Before prescribing ADHD medication for children younger than six, parent training in behavior management should be attempted as the first line of treatment.

Parents who receive training in behavior therapy gain the knowledge, abilities, and methods necessary to assist their kid who has ADHD in achieving success in a variety of settings, including the classroom, the home, and interpersonal connections. The learning and use of behavior therapy is a time- and labor-intensive process, but it yields long-term advantages for both the kid and the family.

The average number of sessions a parent goes through with a therapist is eight or more. During sessions, participants may work independently with a group of parents or a single family. The therapist maintains regular contact with the parents to monitor their development, offer support, and, if necessary, make adjustments to treatment plans to facilitate growth. In most cases, parents must continue practicing with their children between sessions.

Their parents mostly shape the conduct of a young child during the early years. Because young children do not have the maturity to change their behavior without their parent's assistance, the only therapy advised for young children diagnosed with ADHD is a therapy that focuses on training parents. Play therapy and talk therapy are two methods that some therapists may use to treat young children who have ADHD. Children are allowed to talk about their thoughts and feelings through play in the context of play therapy. Talk therapy is a treatment for mental and emotional illnesses involving verbal dialogue between the treated child and a therapist. It has not been demonstrated that either will alleviate symptoms in young children with ADHD.

It takes time and effort to learn and practice behavior therapy, but the child will reap long-term benefits from participating in the therapy. To learn more about the benefits of parent training in behavior treatment for young children with ADHD, talk to your healthcare practitioner.

Behavior Therapy with Children

Psychological therapy aims to treat a mental health illness or assist a kid in managing their symptoms to function effectively at home, school, and in their community. It can also help a child control their symptoms so that they can treat themselves.

It is normal practice for therapists to involve the child's parents when the child is still young. There are occasions when therapists only interact with the parents. Older children have the option of seeing a therapist on their own. Working with the child's entire family or with other significant adults in the child's life is an integral part of certain types of therapy (for example, a teacher).

In most cases, parent-focused techniques involve the parents having a conversation with the therapist about how the child is behaving and how they are feeling. Talking, playing, or engaging in other activities with children as part of psychological treatment can help facilitate the child's expression of their feelings and thoughts. In addition, therapists may monitor interactions between parents and children as a group, after which they may offer suggestions for discovering alternative ways to react.

Approaches using behavior therapy and cognitive-behavior therapy are more likely to reduce symptoms for the most common childhood conditions, such as ADHD, behavior disorders, anxiety, or depression; however, there is limited information about which type of therapy is best for treating each distinct mental disorder that can affect children.

Parents should also be able to do the following;

- Make a habit out of it. Make it a point to stick to the same daily routine, from when you get up to when you go to sleep.
- Get your act together. To reduce the likelihood that your child may misplace their belongings, such as school bags, clothing, and toys, encourage them to keep them in the same spot every day.
- Manage distractions. When your child is working on their schoolwork, ensure the television is turned off, there is as little noise as possible, and the workplace is tidy. Some children who have ADHD can learn better when they are moving around or

listening to music in the background. Keep an eye on your kid, and see what seems to work.

- Limit selections. To prevent your child from becoming overloaded or overstimulated, provide choices from which there are only a few possibilities. For instance, you could ask them to decide between wearing this suit or that one, eating this meal or that one, or playing with this toy or that one.
- When you are speaking with your child, make sure to be explicit and specific. Give your child the impression that you are paying attention by retelling what you overheard them saying. When they have to do anything, use concise and unambiguous directions.
- Assist your child in making plans. Convert laborious activities into easier ones that may be completed in fewer stages. Getting an early start and taking frequent breaks might help reduce stress when working on lengthy projects.
- Make use of goals, praise, and other forms of reward. You can let your child know they have done well by either telling them or rewarding their efforts in various ways after using a chart to establish goals and track positive behaviors. The chart can be found here. Make sure the goals are attainable; remember that taking baby steps is vital!
- Efficiently apply discipline. Due to incorrect behavior, effective directives, time-outs, or the withdrawal of privileges should be used rather than reprimanding, yelling at, or spanking the child.
- Create favorable opportunities. Children who have ADHD could find some circumstances to be upsetting. Discovering and supporting your child's strengths, whether in academics, extracurricular activities, the arts, music, or play, can assist in developing pleasant experiences for the child.

Medical Interventions
Children who take medication for ADHD are better able to manage the symptoms of the condition in their day-to-day lives and are also better able to regulate the behaviors that go in the way of their relationships with their families, friends, and teachers.

- **Stimulants**: are the ADHD treatments with the most name recognition and patient usage. When children with ADHD take these drugs that work quickly, between 70 and 80 percent of them experience a reduction in the severity of their condition.

- **Non-stimulants**: were given the green light for treating ADHD in 2003. Although they do not function as soon as stimulants, their effects might remain in the body for up to twenty-four hours.

Both stimulants and non-stimulants have been given the go-ahead by the Food and Drug Administration (FDA) to assist in lessening the symptoms of attention deficit hyperactivity disorder (ADHD) and enhance functioning in children as young as six years old.

According to Farchione, it may appear contradictory, but stimulants, which contain various forms of methylphenidate and amphetamine, have a calming impact on hyperactive children with ADHD. This is because stimulants contain various versions of these substances. Dopamine is a neurotransmitter associated with motivation, attention, and movement. It is thought that they boost the levels of dopamine in the brain.

Strattera (atomoxetine), Intuniv (guanfacine), and Kapvay are the three non-stimulant treatments for ADHD that the FDA has given its approval to treat the symptoms of the disorder (clonidine). Children who do not respond well to the effects of stimulants may find that these offer a helpful alternative. Discuss with your child's primary caregiver the medications that might work best for your child.

Some children who have ADHD also undergo behavioral therapy in addition to medication to assist in the management of symptoms and to teach additional coping skills. In addition, worried parents can get information and help on how to deal with the symptoms of ADHD by contacting the schools where their children are enrolled and community support groups in their area. "When it comes to managing the disease, engaging with the various individuals involved in a kid's life is helpful.

Brain Training Programs

Brain training as a treatment option for ADHD is becoming increasingly popular and accessible. Programs are available for various devices, including smartphones, desktops, and tablets. Many brain training systems claim they can help typical executive functioning difficulties in persons with ADHD. These difficulties include issues with attention, impulsivity, and working memory. Many applications feature interfaces designed to appear and feel like video games, but their primary purpose is to train particular brain processes.

Both neurofeedback training, which aims to alter physiological activity by monitoring brain waves, and cognitive training, which focuses on improving specific brain skills such as problem-solving and reading comprehension primarily through games and other exercises, are the general categories under which the programs fall. Neurofeedback training has the goal of altering physiological activity.

However, research on whether or not cognitive training can successfully alleviate the symptoms of ADHD is still in its infancy. Several studies have shown that users experience improvements in their brain functioning. However, many question just how much consumers are benefiting from the service. For some patients, neurofeedback can result in increased attention, decreased hyperactivity, and enhanced executive skills, including working memory, according to the research done so far. On the other hand, a number of the most prominent academics working in the field of ADHD believe that the efficacy of neurofeedback in treating ADHD has not been demonstrated beyond a reasonable doubt. The research support for stimulant drug and behavior therapy is stronger than neurofeedback. This is the bottom line.

Music Therapy

It has the potential to improve one's attention as well as their social skills. It has both a rhythm and a structure. In addition, making music demands different regions of your brain to collaborate and teach you how to function effectively within a group setting.

There is very little concrete research that specifically connects music with the symptoms of ADHD. However, researchers do know that when children play an instrument — for example, taking piano lessons at home or playing cello with a school orchestra — they perform significantly better on tests of executive function than children who do not study music. This is the case regardless of whether or not they have ADHD. This refers to the brain's capacity to organize information easily and switch gears between tasks.

If your child would rather kick a soccer ball than pick up a flute, or if they can't sit still for lessons or practice, your child may be able to calm down enough to accomplish their homework if they listen to their favorite playlist. Dopamine, a hormone that assists with focus, is released into your brain when you listen to music that you enjoy and find rewarding.

Even if more research needs to be done to establish a link between ADHD and music, this is undeniably a field that should be investigated, particularly by families who like listening to music.

HOW TO HELP YOUR CHILD MAKE FRIENDS AND IMPROVE SOCIAL SKILLS

Every day, we connect and communicate with the people around us, which requires us to have social skills. We can accomplish this by utilizing verbal and non-verbal modes, specifically eye contact, facial expressions, and body language (volume, speed, tone of voice).

Children diagnosed with Attention-Deficit/Hyperactivity Disorder (ADHD) may have difficulty comprehending and putting various social skills into practice due to their condition. Because of the impairment in their brain's executive functioning, they may have a more difficult time making and maintaining friendships.

The brain's executive control system manages a person's capacity to wait their turn, avoid becoming distracted, coordinate their activities, control their emotions, and use their working memory to respond appropriately in social situations. Children who have ADHD may have a delay in the development of their executive functions, up to thirty percent longer than their classmates.

In social situations, symptoms of ADHD might involve a variety of different things, such as;

Inattentive
- Difficulty listening to others
- Missing pieces of information
- Being distracted by sounds or noises
- Missing social cues
- Becoming overwhelmed and withdrawn

Hyperactive
- Frequently interrupting
- Sharing scattered thoughts
- Being hyper-focused on a topic
- Talking rapidly or excessively

Impulsive
- Goofy behavior at inappropriate times
- Entering others' personal space
- Displaying aggression
- Initiating conversations at inappropriate times

Children who have ADHD may have difficulty sharing, taking turns, listening, and picking up on social cues when they are in a social context. This can be frustrating for everyone involved. They frequently show signs of boredom, become sidetracked, or otherwise disengage from the conversation. When engaging with their classmates, children with ADHD may find it challenging to maintain control of their feelings. They may quickly get overwhelmed, lose their patience, or become frustrated.

When children with ADHD become distracted in social interactions or take the lead in the topic, their classmates may regard them as indifferent and unpleasant. This is especially true if children with ADHD tend to dominate the conversation. These children's peers will most likely steer clear of them. Because of this, they miss out on opportunities to develop their social skills, leading to a decline in their confidence in their abilities. Children will begin to feel inadequacy and develop unfavorable emotional responses to other people's behaviors if they do not have social relationships. Some children with ADHD may even shun all social interactions to protect themselves from being teased or bullied, even worse.

They must have adequate social functioning and good peer interactions to reach their full potential. Children acquire the skills necessary to collaborate, negotiate, and find solutions to problems with other people when they have positive experiences interacting with their peers. They can cultivate fruitful relationships with their contemporaries due to these qualities. As a result, social supports are factors that promote protection. They give a person a feeling of acceptance, purpose, belonging, and a sense that they are cared for. When children reach the age of puberty, they have a greater demand for social engagement with their peers and a heightened sensitivity to the various social cues that surround them. Friendships are formed through regular social encounters, which teach teenagers how to work in a group, solve problems, identify the points of view of others, handle peer conflict, and embrace varied groups of people.

Children with attention deficit hyperactivity disorder (ADHD) may have difficulty interpreting social cues and efficiently practicing social skills. The following aspects of social functioning may be impaired due to the condition: listening to others, beginning discussions at the proper times, frequently interrupting, failing to pick up on social cues, retreating, and talking excessively. These difficulties can affect relationships in everyday settings such as schools, homes, and communities. The quality and number of opportunities to practice social skills have drastically decreased due to the pandemic. Even while these challenges will not go away, parents may help their children comprehend and develop their social skills by providing them with opportunities at home.

Below Are Tips to Help Your Child Improve Social Skills
Some skills are quantifiable during development—language, math, etc. But what about the more nebulous abilities, such as social skills, that don't come as naturally to people? Children who have ADHD sometimes have a difficult time developing friends and keeping existing ties. There are a lot of parents that are curious about how to teach their children social skills, but most of them are clueless about where to begin. Activities geared toward social skills development and other methods that, when combined, can help your child feel more confident in their abilities are included in our list of eight ways.

Rehearse Acceptable Responses
The symptoms of ADHD in children are not often obvious, particularly to the child's peers. Because they do not communicate in the same way that other children do, many children who have ADHD are misunderstood, and this difference can be problematic for the children with whom they are enrolled in school. Your child can learn acceptable alternatives to impolite or harsh statements by practicing them in rehearsal, which is a wonderful approach to teaching them. During this time, you should also emphasize keeping eye contact and having a relaxed body posture.

Observe and Intervene
Your child's present skill set can be better understood if you see them interact with other children during play dates. At any point throughout the play date, you should be prepared to step in and help your child if they are having difficulty. If your child makes a disrespectful remark, you should quickly offer more acceptable alternatives to assist them in becoming more mature.

Encourage Peer - Pairs at School
When it comes to projects and other assignments, many teachers put students in groups. Children who have ADHD can hone their social skills through participation in collaborative projects like these. Have

a conversation with your kid's educator and find out if they can incorporate more group projects into the classroom.

Encourage Friendship At Home

Children who have ADHD may feel more at ease interacting with others when they are at home because this environment is more familiar to them. You should host a pizza night, complete with your child's pals, where they can bring games, watch movies, and eat pizza. In an environment in which your child is already at ease, you are in the best position to observe, guide, and model acceptable social conduct for them.

Wait For Cues

Children are more likely to respond positively to helpful counsel at the appropriate time. Wait till your child has calmed down and expressed their emotions before delivering it to them. This will make them more receptive to what you have to say after a heated disagreement or similar event that they have experienced.

Improve Your Relationship With Your Child

Children who have healthy relationships with both of their parents are more likely to have positive outcomes in terms of their social development. Parents need to make plans to spend quality time with their children on multiple occasions each week. During this time, you should refrain from bringing up any ADHD symptoms. Instead, it would be best to concentrate on having fun and developing a closer relationship with your child.

Build On Your Child's Interest

If your child is interested in a certain activity, you should promote that interest to build their self-confidence. Children who have ADHD may find that participating in group activities such as team sports or art classes is particularly beneficial.

Lead By Example

You may be confident that your child will pick up on and improve their social skills if you set a good example for them. In addition, you can also mention to the parents of other children that your child has difficulties interacting with other children socially. When they better understand the circumstances, they may be more inclined to set up playdates and other enjoyable activities.

Children of all ages need healthy friendships and relationships with their peers. Unfortunately, many children who have attention deficit hyperactivity disorder (ADHD) struggle to make and maintain friendships, as well as to be accepted by their more general peer group. The symptoms of attention deficit hyperactivity disorder (ADHD), which include impulsivity, hyperactivity, and inattention, can wreak havoc on a child's attempts to interact with others in healthy ways.

It is possible that not being accepted by one's peer group, feeling alienated, different, unlikeable, and alone is the most painful element of ADHD-related impairments, and the impacts of these experiences can continue for a long time. Building healthy relationships with other people is of the utmost significance. Even while children who have ADHD have a strong desire to socialize and be accepted by their peers, they frequently lack the skills necessary to do so. The encouraging news is that you can play a role in assisting your child in the development of these social skills and abilities so they can relate well with friends.

Increase Your Child's Social Awareness
Children who have ADHD typically have a very difficult time monitoring their behavior in social settings. They frequently do not have a good comprehension of social settings or awareness of the reactions they generate in others. They might believe that a conversation they had with a peer went well, for instance, even when it was obvious that it did not. Difficulties associated with ADHD can lead to deficiencies in a person's ability to analyze or "read" a social situation effectively and in their capacity to self-evaluate, self-monitor, and change as required. Your child needs to get instruction from you directly for these abilities.

Teach Skills And How To Relate Directly
Children with ADHD typically struggle to draw meaningful conclusions from their past experiences. They frequently act without giving any thought to the possible outcomes. These children can be helped in several ways, one of which is by receiving rapid and regular criticism regarding social faux pas or inappropriate behavior. Playing roles is a great approach to teaching, modeling, and practicing positive social skills and different ways to react in difficult situations, such as when someone teases you.

Your first step should be zero in on the one or two areas in which your child has the most difficulty. This helps to ensure that the learning process does not become too overwhelming.

Many children who have ADHD struggle with basic skills, such as initiating and maintaining a conversation, interacting with some other person fairly and equitably (for example, listening, asking questions about the other child's ideas or feelings, taking turns in the discussion, or expressing interest in the other child), negotiating and settling disputes as they emerge, sharing, sustaining personal space, and even actually talking in a normal tone of voice that is not too loud.

Your child should be aware of the social rules you want them to follow and the behaviors you want to see from them, and you should provide them with information on these topics. Repeatedly working on these abilities can help you become a better member of society. Motivate desirable activities through the provision of instant gratification

Create Opportunities For Friendship Development

Play dates are an excellent opportunity for preschool and elementary school parents to coach and model positive peer interactions for their children. They are also an excellent opportunity for the child to practice the new skills they have learned. Instead of organizing these playdates for a large group of your child's pals, you should organize them for only one or two friends at a time. Playtime should be organized to maximize your child's chances of success.

Consider yourself your child's "relationship coach" in this situation. When planning a playdate for your child, it is important to consider how long the event will go and select activities that will keep your child interested the entire time.

It is often the case that a child's friendships and relationships with their peers become more challenging as they get older, yet, it is equally crucial for you to continue being involved and foster positive interactions between peers. The years spent in middle and high school can be quite challenging for a child with difficulty interacting with others. Even if the peer group does not accept a child as a whole during their formative years, having is not accepted by the peer group as a whole throughout their formative years, having at least one supportive friend throughout this time can frequently shield the child from the full-blown negative impacts that come along with being shunned by their peers.

Students in middle or high school who have been socially isolated and repeatedly rejected may feel anxious to belong to any peer group that would accept them, even if that group negatively influences them.

Do some research on the organizations in your town, such as the Boy Scouts, Indian Guides, Girl Scouts, Girls on the Run, and sports teams that encourage the development of strong peer relationships and social skills, and get involved with some of those organizations. Check if the people in charge of the group or the coaches are aware of attention deficit hyperactivity disorder (ADHD) and can foster a helpful and encouraging atmosphere for developing prosocial skills.

Maintain open lines of communication with your child's school, their coaches, and the other parents in the neighborhood so that you are aware of what is going on with your child and who they are spending time with. A child's circle of friends and the qualities shared by those friends significantly impact the development of the children who are part of that circle.

Work With The Child's School To Improve Peer Status

Suppose a child's peer group negatively labels them because of deficiencies in social skills. In that case, it can be very difficult for that child to shed this reputation after it has been established. A poor reputation is likely one of your child's most significant challenges when interacting with others.

Studies have shown that the negative peer status of children with ADHD is often already established by the early to middle elementary school years, and this reputation can stick with the child even as they begin to make positive changes in social skills. One possible explanation for this phenomenon is that children with ADHD are more hyperactive and impulsive than their typically developing peers. For this reason, it can be important for parents to work with the teachers, coaches, and other adults their children interact with regularly to address these reputational impacts.

Develop a productive working connection with the educator caring for your child. Share with them your child's strengths and interests and the challenges they've recently faced in their development. Please provide any approaches you have discovered to be effective when working on your child's areas of difficulty.

When young children acquire social preferences about their friends, they frequently seek their instructors for guidance. The warmth, patience, and acceptance can influence a child's social standing and the gentle redirection they receive from a teacher. This can act as a model for the child's peer group.

When a child has been unsuccessful in the classroom, it becomes even more necessary for the teacher to find ways to draw positive attention to that child intentionally. This attention should be given to acknowledge the child's previous struggles. One strategy for accomplishing this goal is to give the child in question unique responsibilities and assignments while the other students in the classroom are watching them.

Make sure that these are responsibilities your child can complete, which will help them build improved emotions of self-worth and acceptance from their peers in the classroom. This not only gives the peer group opportunities to view your child from a good perspective, but it can also help stop the group process of peer rejection. It may also be helpful to place the child in the company of a sympathetic "buddy" in the school. This can speed up the process of gaining social acceptability.

Work with your child's teacher to make the classroom as "ADHD-friendly" as possible so your child will have an easier time controlling the symptoms of ADHD. This will help your child succeed in school. Collaborate with the classroom instructor, as well as with the coach or any other adult caregiver, to develop strategies for effective behavior control and instruction in social skills.

TECHNIQUES TO HELP YOUR CHILD HANDLE INTENSE EMOTIONS WITHOUT THROWING A TANTRUM

Children who have ADHD experience the same emotions as people who do not have the illness. There are many different emotions, such as happiness, rage, fear, and sadness. Their feelings are more intense, they persist for a longer period, and they experience them more frequently. They frequently have an effect on life in general as well.

When you're a parent or a caretaker for a child, it might be challenging to comprehend the reasons behind their behavior. You may think they're just trying to be difficult. However, it is essential to keep in mind that they are not acting intentionally in this manner. It may take them longer and require more work to learn how to manage their conduct. Here is the information that you require.

Many children behave without thinking things through or become overly excited to the point where they have trouble cooling down. They typically outgrow this phase as they mature and acquire the ability to control their feelings. This is referred to as self-regulation. Specialists have compared the situation to that of a thermostat, which is activated to maintain the desired temperature in the room. When your child's feelings go out of control, they will learn to take their own "temperature" and calm themselves down.

Children who have ADHD often struggle to control their emotions, which can lead to meltdowns, outbursts, and other problematic behaviors. Please find out how parents can serve as emotional role models for their children and contribute to creating supportive surroundings in this book.

Emotional regulation abilities, often called self-regulatory skills, allow us to handle challenging situations and feelings without being unduly triggered or spinning out of control. The intense emotional reactivity that can be a symptom of attention deficit hyperactivity disorder (ADHD or ADD), a condition that impairs executive functioning and, as a result, affects our ability to manage attention, time, and emotions effectively, can be just as disruptive as almost any other symptom.

Outbursts, meltdowns, and tantrums are strong emotional bouts that are intimately recognizable to the parents of children with ADHD. These extreme emotional bouts leave the parent and the kid feeling tired and possibly powerless. What they might not realize is that children with ADHD can be taught the skills necessary to regulate their emotions through a combination of behavioral therapies, awareness training, medication, and mindfulness practices.

Strategy 1: Accurate label feelings

Emotional intelligence is the capacity to be aware of, express, and manage our emotions on our own and in the context of our relationships. Effective emotional regulation is dependent on emotional intelligence. The first step in this process is to become aware of our sentiments as they shift and change, which is not as simple as it may sound.

A more complex emotional lexicon enriches our experiences of feeling different emotions. If you know "anger," you will label any other feeling related to anger as "anger." You will be able to pinpoint your experience with greater precision if you can detect, in a more understated manner, when you feel "annoyed," "anxious," "sad," "frustrated," or "disappointed." How we make sense of challenging experiences can change depending on the size of our emotional toolkit.

A family accepting of all feelings is the foundation for a healthy emotional acquaintance. Ignoring one's feelings isn't going to get you very far because they all have a purpose. Therefore there's not much point in doing so. For instance, being angry might keep us safe in some situations, while being sad can indicate to those around you that you require help. Emotional maturity comes with age. Thus it's natural for younger children to struggle with handling difficult emotions. Read stories to your child, have conversations about how people feel, and explain how you are feeling.

Help children feel comfortable expressing their feelings by talking openly about them and modeling healthy coping strategies. You may say, "I'm angry; let's discuss once I've calmed down." It is wise to practice emotional self-control every once in a while. Your child does not necessarily need to know how worried or furious they make you. However, when you can do so, demonstrating emotional self-control is a teaching tool in and of itself for children.

Even so, a household that is emotionally open does not, of course, eliminate all of life's difficulties. When a child struggles with their feelings, it is not the parents' fault; rather, this is frequently a symptom of ADHD in and of itself.

Strategy 2: Behavior interventions

For children with difficulties, behavioral treatments are a labor-intensive but proven method for improving their emotional skills. Behavioral programs are essential to the educational process, even for the most well-behaved child. While some programs deal directly with children, others teach parents how to support their children better.

Child-directed treatment, in which children learn to identify their feelings first and then acquire coping skills to deal with what they are experiencing, can be extremely helpful for adults and children with attention deficit hyperactivity disorder (ADHD). The involvement of parents is beneficial because adults may emphasize what their children might otherwise neglect to work on without their aid. While learning to manage their disruptive emotions, therapy focusing on children should guide them in forming useful new habits.

On the other hand, one helpful short-term method for mood management is often entirely dependent on the parents' actions. What we know about how the brain develops is reflected in behavioral parent training (BPT), which teaches young children to learn primarily through instant feedback. Recognizing the distinction between our feelings and actions is one of the most fundamental lessons that can be learned from BPT. Parents should make it their mission to validate their children's feelings, not the undesirable behaviors they exhibit: "I can understand that you are upset, but it is never OK to hit." Successfully managing children's emotions requires a well-coordinated behavioral strategy that strikes a balance between positive reinforcement (such as praise and rewards) and strict boundaries (such as limitations and punishments).

Tantrums, for instance, are frequently nothing more than a behavior provoked by a cause. "I don't want to stop playing my video game" is an example of such a cause. This makes sense; we all get irritated. We affirm that anger through a behavioral plan by saying things like "I realize that you're frustrated," but we also link it to more proper conduct by saying things like "If you shut down your game responsibly, you can have 15 more minutes tomorrow." The takeaway from this is that all feelings are acceptable, but certain behaviors are not.

Treatment for ADHD that is based on research includes behavioral programs. However, many people give up on them too soon since getting them to function properly may require much painstaking effort and customization. Continue making modifications until you find a successful tactic, and if your method does not appear to be working, speak with an expert or a trainer.

Strategy 3: ADHD Medication
Many people can treat their medical conditions without needing medicine, which is wonderful when it's successful. However, there are occasions when our bodies want more. Because of this, it's possible that medicine can play a big part in helping individuals with ADHD better regulate their emotions.

ADD, and ADHD are both medical conditions. Although this does not imply that medication is the sole tool available to cope with it, it does legitimize the consideration of medication as an option. When prescribed and taken in the recommended manner, medicines for ADHD are both safe and effective. Despite the widespread misunderstandings, the appropriate drug should have advantages while having no substantial adverse effects.

Although drugs for ADHD are not designed to address emotional reactivity, many people find that they are helpful in this area. It is important to keep a close eye on your child's symptoms while you are making adjustments to their medication for attention deficit hyperactivity disorder (ADHD) because these medications can either improve or worsen irritability. Collaborate with your healthcare provider to determine the appropriate dosage and medication for your child until you reach a point where you are at ease with the treatment they are receiving.

When choosing medicine for ADHD, the clinician needs to consider whether the patient also has another ailment at the same time. One, such as anxiety or a sleep disturbance, is present in as many as two-thirds of children diagnosed with ADHD. In some cases, emotional symptoms can be caused by these diseases, even in the absence of ADHD.

Strategy 4: Mindfulness meditation
The practice of mindfulness involves bringing one's full, undivided attention to the here-and-now circumstances, regardless of whether or not those circumstances are positive or negative. To be quite clear, the premise does not state that we will always be tranquil or cheerful. The only way to successfully navigate the ever-shifting

landscape of life is to arm yourself with the abilities necessary to do so.

One of the most well-established advantages of practicing mindfulness is that it helps people better control their emotions. It works as a muscle trainer for our brain as time goes on. We can hard-wire new characteristics, such as observing discomfort without reacting immediately. The discipline of recognizing feelings allows us to avoid getting into the routine habits that we all have.

Most of us spend significant time distracted, acting impulsively, and operating on autopilot. For instance, if our child throws another fit, we may experience exhaustion and succumb to mindless routines, such as giving in to their demands or employing excessively severe punishments. But as we practice mindfulness, our capacity to remain calm increases, enabling us to see our alternatives more clearly and take action with a more defined purpose.

The practice of mindfulness is most frequently accomplished through meditation. During this practice, we focus on objectives, such as the sensation of our breath or the contact of our feet with the ground, so we always have a point of reference to return to when our busy minds wander. As soon as there is another thing to distract us, we will begin again. By doing so, we form a new pattern of awareness and learn to manage our feelings effectively.

When it comes to families, practicing mindfulness should start with the adults. While we tend to react emotionally to situations more quickly than we should, it is not very helpful to advise others, such as our children, to practice mindfulness. As another unavoidable aspect of life, the cycle of anger and reactivity inevitably leads to even more anger, and reactivity cannot be avoided. If you model mindful living for your children, they will pick up the practice more easily.

Introduce your children to mindfulness whenever you have the chance; this could take the form of a little meditation before bedtime for smaller children or the search for a teen group for older children. The overarching objective is to establish the seeds that will one day lead to a consistent mindfulness practice for your children. This is true even if your child is initially resistant to the idea.

The practice of mindfulness eventually becomes second nature. We become aware of what is occurring on the inside ("I am so furious") and make room for decisions that are more beneficial to our health ("I'm going to quiet down before I figure out what to do"). Recent research, which should come as no surprise, reveals that children with ADHD, some of whom are as young as seven years old, can get unique benefits for managing their emotions.

Temper tantrums, wrath, and emotionality are all symptoms of ADHD, and they all contribute to an increase in stress, a decrease in positive connections, and overall difficulty in life. The habit, in turn, undermines the resiliency that is necessary to handle ADHD in the first place, which further escalates the emotions of everyone involved. There are even repercussions for one's health: Intense and chronic tantrums make it more difficult to encourage children to eat, sleep, or even exercise, undermining parents' ability to regulate their children's emotions. Multiple advantages can be gained by learning to rein in one's anger and other negative emotions.

Strategy 5: Preempt the emotion

These first two abilities are meant to be utilized here and now while the feeling has taken control. On the other hand, in the long run, it is important to recognize patterns and warning indications before an outburst occurs. Invest some time in monitoring your child so that you may obtain a sense of the common triggers that they experience. You may be able to head off big escalations in emotion by doing this. For instance, if your kid tends to get "hangry," you should postpone challenging chats until after he's had something to eat.

Strategy 6: Raise self-awareness

Additionally, it is beneficial for children to learn how to "develop the muscle" of being able to tolerate harsh emotions; however, this process should gradually occur. Work with your kid during times of peace to help her recognize when she is most likely to become upset and how she may tell when her feelings are beginning to rise. What sensations does she have throughout her body? What kinds of things does she have running through her mind? When children become familiar with the signals they exhibit of emotional arousal, they can practice the skills necessary for self-regulation before it is too late. These include taking slow, deep breaths, visualizing happy or uplifting scenes in their minds, or physically removing themselves from a stressful situation. With practice, these abilities will eventually become second nature, and she will develop a greater capacity for independently initiating procedures for self-regulation.

Strategy 7: Model self-regulation skills

Children pick up information about feelings from the people in their immediate environment. The more you can bring your feelings under control, the more they will be able to learn to do the same for themselves. Your child may still be able to observe your distress despite this fact. The realization that it is okay for them to have these sensations (at safe levels) and that there is something that they can do about it is extremely beneficial to children. When you are unhappy, it is healthy to let your emotions appear in tiny doses, to talk about your feelings using language suitable for your developmental level, and, most importantly, to talk about what you are going to do to help yourself feel calmer. Young children will look forward to participating with you in activities that promote self-regulation, such as the ones listed above, and it will be beneficial for them to get into the habit of doing so.

Strategy 8: Build your tolerance for their distress

It is normal for children to exhibit extreme responses when confronted with powerful emotions when they are still mastering the skill of self-regulation. The hope is to instill a sense of self-assurance in their capacity to self-soothe, but this cannot be accomplished immediately. When your child is having a meltdown, remind yourself that he is doing the best he can at that moment and that once he has regained his composure, you can continue to work with him to build the muscles he needs to regulate his emotions. Take a few deep breaths and have faith that if you can stay regulated in those most difficult moments, it will help your child see that he is safe and protected by you even when he doesn't feel safe and protected in his own body. Take a few deep breaths and have faith that if you can stay regulated in those most difficult of moments, it will help your child see that he is safe and protected by you. And don't forget to reassure yourself that you, too, are working hard! Everyone has to put in a lot of effort to learn how to self-regulate. It will grow less difficult as time goes by!

Targeting future-oriented prosocial emotions is particularly important for children with ADHD because they live in the moment and cannot think ahead about the consequences of their emotions or behaviors. As a result, targeting future-oriented prosocial emotions is particularly important for these children. Children with ADHD benefit greatly from cultivating future-oriented prosocial feelings such as gratitude, pride, and compassion because doing so helps them establish tenacity, cooperation, and empathy. Listed below are some tried-and-true methods for constructing them:

Six Ways to Cultivate Gratitude

Being thankful can protect us from emotional "overreactions" and help us develop the ability to defer gratification. When we feel grateful for what we already have, it causes us to cease looking for what we perceive to be the next greatest thing. Here are some suggestions that can help you develop thankfulness.

- Always remember to be grateful. Establish a family tradition, such as sharing the five things you are grateful for each day or sharing what inspired you today. This may be a fun way to bond with one another.
- Make a thankfulness jar. Because of the visual nature of ADHD, it may be helpful for children to "see" the emotion of thankfulness if they regularly write letters of thanks.
- Urge them to compose handwritten notes of gratitude to you. Remembering all the significant individuals in our lives is integral to practicing gratitude. It would be best if you encouraged your child to express gratitude to those who have assisted them over the week by sending thank-you notes.
- Create a tribal tree of support as step number four. Please give them a piece of paper or poster board, and have them decorate it in the shape of a tree. Then, have them write the names of people in their lives who are supportive of them, such as family members, friends, teachers, coaches, youth ministers, and so on. They should display the tree in a visible location to serve as a constant reminder of all the people who have been there for them.
- Establish a System of Reciprocal Assistance. Someone who requires assistance with something, such as schoolwork or another form of activity, will write the "job" they need help with on a Post-It note or whiteboard. Imagine that it's an ad for family members looking for assistance. The name of the assistant is then written down on the paper. The many family members may understand, in an easily digestible format, how each other contributes to their well-being. It is proven that helping others improves our mood. Displaying these acts of generosity helps to build a spirit of cooperation and collaboration within the family, which is essential to maintaining harmonious relationships.
- Compose some "I Noticed" Notes. Because children with ADHD are subjected to so much constructive criticism throughout a typical day, they need to observe and acknowledge instances of kindness.

Notes beginning with "I Noticed" are an excellent method for drawing attention to prosocial conduct and offering an ongoing stream of positive feedback, which assists children and adolescents with ADHD to remain on track. Because someone has taken time out of their day to produce a hand-written note, they can foster feelings of gratitude in the recipient.

Three ways to build pride

Even more so than motivation, self-efficacy, self-esteem, or even being pleased, pride is a goal-directed feeling that directly encourages self-control, effort, and perseverance. When we feel proud of ourselves, it inspires us to put more effort into our tasks. Connection and contribution are the two most important factors in developing pride. Children need to have the sense that they are contributing something worthwhile to the lives of those who are significant to them.

- Give your child the opportunity to become an expert in anything that captures their interest. Dog walker. Video game master. Cleaner for the bathroom sink. It doesn't even make a difference. The most important thing is to identify an area in which the child excels and provide them with opportunities to teach others using those areas of expertise. Allow them to weigh in on significant matters that also pertain to their expertise.
- Give your child a task that they will find meaningful. Even if you can do it a third of the time and with a tenth of the mess, the answer is still yes. Keep an eye out for those with fundamental life skills such as making scrambled eggs or ironing a cotton shirt. When children can make significant contributions to the family, not only do the children profit but so do their parents. When children believe they are contributing to the group, it motivates them to work harder on challenging tasks, even if they do the work independently. They could be able to finish a chore (like pumping up the bike tires, for example) that will help the family go on a bike ride together, such as preparing the bikes for the ride. Play positive music for them or offer encouragement when working through a challenging assignment. This will help motivate them to get through the challenge.
- Make a skills board. Please make a list of their strengths and the qualities that people admire, such as their ability to reassure young children or their thoughtfulness when others are in pain.

Five ways to help your child act with compassion

Compassion is a vitally important prosocial emotion that assists in overcoming anxiety, avoidance, and procrastination while encouraging empathy and cooperation.

- Consider your family a unit you should lead. The most effective method for fostering compassion is to highlight shared experiences. Any hint will do, even something as simple as dressing alike. Because of this, all of the athletes in a team wear the same shirt. It brings them closer together as a unit. You and your family may volunteer to clean up a public outdoor spot together. Everyone should wear the T-shirts made especially for the event on the specified Saturday. Compassion can be fostered in individuals through various activities, including collaboratively pursuing a common objective, exchanging information about topics of mutual interest, recognizing and celebrating one another's accomplishments, and providing support to one another.
- Play a game like "Never Have I Ever" to get people talking to one another. Every participant takes turns to question the others about activities they haven't participated in. For example, "I've never fractured my arm." If a participant in the game has suffered a broken arm, the score is kept on a piece of paper. Continue playing until everyone has had an opportunity to contribute. Children benefit from experiences like these because it helps them see the myriad ways they are connected to others.
- Meditation that focuses on the present moment. Meditation was first used in ancient times by Buddhist monks to cultivate compassion; this practice, which dates back hundreds of years, is still effective today. There are a lot of applications that assist you through meditation, but it's not hard to create opportunities to practice being in the here and now, such as by paying attention to the sights, sounds, and sensations you encounter when walking around your area.
- Encourage children to be kind to themselves by teaching them self-compassion. Children who have ADHD receive a lot of corrective input, and as a result, they frequently experience feelings of guilt and shame. As a result, these children need to have compassion for themselves. Self-compassion gives people the ability to acknowledge and accept their shortcomings, including the reality that having ADHD may need them to put in more effort than other people in certain situations. In the early stages, an excellent strategy to cultivate self-compassion is to have conversations about

neurodiversity and everyone's talents and weaknesses. In the same way that I need glasses to see as far as other people, they may require additional time to calm down after recess before they can focus on learning. When discussing one's strengths and shortcomings, it is important to highlight the positive aspects of having ADHD, such as having an abundance of energy or being incredibly creative.

- Explain to them how their brain works. It is helpful to teach children about their brains, specifically how they are still evolving and how they may help build their brains through things like diet, sleep, and coping skills. Then, for instance, when kids get distracted, they understand that their brains became too excited by the sound in the corridor, and they can figure out what they need to do to get their brains back on track and continue focusing on what they were doing before they became distracted (vs. internalizing I am stupid).

Explore a variety of approaches to teaching your child the values of appreciation, pride, and compassion in their daily lives. Keep in mind that children are always developing. Likewise, your family's methods to cultivate positive mental attitudes to gain emotional control will do the same. Be patient, and remember that nothing can take the place of deliberate practice and thoughtful critique of your performance.

YOUR CHILD'S ADHD SUPERPOWERS AND HOW YOU CAN CULTIVATE THESE QUALITIES IN HIM

The difficulties associated with Attention Deficit Hyperactivity Disorder (ADHD) typically come to mind when the term is brought up. Nevertheless, it is of the utmost need to acknowledge the numerous beneficial elements of ADHD as well. People who have ADHD have a variety of extraordinary abilities, some of which may even appear to be superpowers to those who do not have ADHD; nonetheless, it is essential that people who have ADHD feel empowered to embrace their inner superheroes.

The following is a list of nine incredible ADHD superpowers that will assist you in becoming your superhero and help individuals who may not yet be aware of their abilities.

Endless Energy
Some persons with ADHD can give the impression that they "are always on the move," which may be helpful when attempting to get things done. Because you have an endless supply of energy, you might be an athlete who can play the whole game, still have enough energy left over to hang out with friends afterward, and still have enough energy left over to prepare for the physics test you have the next day. Or, your children with ADHD can spend the entire day playing and still find time to pitch in around the house.

You might also have the ability to "think quickly on your feet," which is a skill that comes in very handy when you are faced with the challenge of choosing how to proceed when faced with a challenging circumstance. This superpower is analogous to the Flash, who can move, think, and run at breakneck speeds.

This can be a terrible nightmare before bed, during extended vehicle drives, or in the middle of class. Make advantage of all this potential energy. It can have tremendous outcomes for your child's ability to focus if you get them to exercise or use up their energy before school.

There should be many more opportunities for your child to move around, including standing desks, lots of body breaks, and more learning that is done through hands-on activities. It is unrealistic to expect children to lead a sedentary lifestyle. Thus they must get plenty of exercise.

Creativity

People with attention deficit hyperactivity disorder (ADHD) tend to exhibit many creative elements of themselves and the ability to think creatively and from a fresh point of view. Your capacity for creativity will serve you well as you traverse the many projects you pursue, whether it is the production of works of art, the composition of poetry, or the creation of a new application. The capacity to creatively design one's technically advanced armor for various purposes, such as the ability to fly, super-strength, and durability, can be compared to the superpower possessed by Iron Man.

Kids are considerably more likely to resist learning by rote and respond much better to hands-on, problem-solving activities where they can be imaginative. Your child's ability to exercise this muscle can be encouraged by providing classroom and home opportunities. This will assist in keeping your child interested and focused.

Novelty

People who have ADHD despise the state of being bored, and as a result, they have an insatiable appetite for the novelty to maintain a sense of excitement in their lives. It's possible that you deliberately seek out new experiences, that you take pleasure in gaining new knowledge, and that you seek out settings that are intriguing and engaging.

Keeping yourself interested in the things you're passionate about can be accomplished by channeling your appetite for variety. In 1941, when the vast majority of comic book superheroes were male, Wonder Woman stood out as a truly original and innovative character because she symbolized the independence of women. She is regarded as a founding member of the Justice League and is thought to possess a level of power comparable to that of Superman, making her deserving of Thor's hammer.

Ability to hyperfocus

People with ADHD have attentional variances, even though ADHD is commonly perceived as a disorder of attentional deficits. You can use hyperfocus or laser focus on a task to the point where you are no longer aware of anything else in your surroundings.

Due to this heightened state of attention and concentration, you can concentrate on a project with such intensity that several hours may pass without your awareness, and it is possible that you will not even realize how much time has passed. This could be analogous to how Superman's laser vision enables him to intensely emit laser beams from his eyes, which can then be used to either melt things or destroy them.

The most effective method for 'hooking' them is to provide them with opportunities to learn stuff in a way that is tailored to their particular areas of interest. When you are attempting to attract their attention or to get them to pull away from the task they are engaged in, letting them know how much time they have left to complete it is an effective strategy. You still have fifteen minutes left to play, Timmy. There will only be 5 minutes left for you to play before you start doing your responsibilities.

Problem-solving

Finding answers to challenges is, at its core, what constitutes the act of problem-solving as an art form. People who have ADHD can think both rapidly and creatively, which makes them excellent problem solvers. This skill allows them to think outside the box.

When it comes to problem-solving and coming up with solutions, the fact that you may be able to look at situations from various perspectives can give you an advantage. This can put you on the same level as Batman regarding your ability to be an exceptional investigator and track down the nefarious criminal responsible for the crimes.

Curiosity

People who have ADHD tend to take pleasure in trying out new experiences, so it seems to be the reason that they would be interested in discovering more about the world around them and would have a natural curiosity about it. Suppose you enjoy disassembling things to figure out how they function or taking pleasure in picking things up to study them more closely. In that case, you are naturally curious about the world around you.

With her enormous and immense sorcery talents, the Scarlet Witch (Wanda Maximoff) pushes the borders of reality and consciousness, which astounds everyone who comes into contact with her.

Charisma

Some people who have ADHD have a unique magnetic charm or attraction about them, which makes it easy for them to attract the attention and admiration of other people. People who have ADHD may have a distinct talent that makes them natural leaders and influencers, and having this power can be advantageous to you in so many different ways as you manage your profession and interact with social media.

As the King of Wakanda, the Black Panther unquestionably exhibited the power of charisma by leading his people with bravery and courage. He was also the embodiment of the Black Panther's name.

Multitasking

Having a diagnosis of ADHD does not necessarily preclude a person from having the ability to perform many tasks at the same time. If you find that you can talk on the phone while also answering emails, all while watching a Marvel Superhero movie, you know how to multitask. The ADHD brain is great at ping-ponging from one thing to another, so if you find that you can do this, you have ADHD. Spiderman was a master multitasker since he had to juggle several different roles, including those of a student, a superhero, a freelance photographer, and even Tony Stark's (Iron Man) personal assistant at times.

Perseverance

This can be defined as the determination to try to do anything even though difficult, and this tenacity is frequently at the core of what individuals with ADHD emanate. You may need to put in twice as much effort as other people to achieve something, and while this may feel extremely discouraging, it can help you develop a strong sense of resolve to keep going until you are successful. She began her life as a penniless orphan, but she worked hard and persisted to become a master of espionage, a terrific assassin, and an amazing martial artist. Black Widow is one of the most formidable heroes in the Marvel Cinematic Universe.

It can be a tremendous blessing to have a high level of sensitivity to other people's feelings and a heightened awareness of their body language, facial expressions, and tone of voice.

Although this can lead to sensory overload, it also gives them a high level of empathy and sensitivity to others, which in turn allows them to have profound insights into the feelings and behaviors of other people.

They are wonderful companions, and they are also effective activists and social workers. They need to be careful that they learn to establish healthy boundaries to avoid the trap of taking on the issues or experiences of other people as if they were their own, and they need to be vigilant that they learn to set appropriate boundaries.

You may help your child discover their incredible superpowers by following the steps described above. To ever be successful in removing these superpowers from your child, you must have an incredible amount of patience, love, care for them, and, most importantly, an understanding heart.

Many parents of children who struggle academically or behaviorally describe having similar superpowers.' The development of individualized education programs (IEPs), the management of behavior at home, and the discovery of what inspires your child can all benefit from your being aware of your child's strengths or "superpowers."

For instance, if your kid has a lot of creative potential, giving them more chances to use that creativity while at school can make a huge difference in how effectively they complete their assigned homework and other schoolwork. It's possible that your kid isn't even aware of the incredible ways they are special. Please spend some time highlighting the times when their superpower is particularly effective.

When I was a teacher, I had a student who had severe dyslexia, and it had a significant negative influence on his self-esteem. Within weeks, I could observe how wise he was and how remarkable his auditory memory was. Because he was always more than happy to assist with duties or chores in the classroom, I made it a point to incorporate opportunities for him to demonstrate his abilities and put them to use.

This had a positive effect on both his sense of self-worth and his overall motivation in the classroom. With this newfound insight, you and your kid will be better able to see this singular diagnosis in a broader context.

THE CRUCIAL ROLE OF ROUTINES IN YOUR CHILD'S DAILY LIFE

We've all been told that having a structure in our homes is beneficial, particularly for children with attention deficit hyperactivity disorder (ADHD). But what precisely do we mean when we talk about structure, and how can we bring it into our family? Put another way, the structure ensures that things are organized and predictable. Our children can better concentrate on one task at a time, which makes day-to-day functioning much more bearable. And this is of utmost significance for children with attention deficit hyperactivity disorder (ADHD) since these kids have a hard time self-regulating and keeping their focus when there are a lot of distractions pushing them in different directions.

Structure in an environment denotes that it is structured and can be anticipated. Every child benefits from having a structure in their lives, but it can be especially helpful for parents raising children with attention deficit hyperactivity disorder (ADHD).

According to the findings of one study, children of all ages, regardless of how old they are, are better able to control their conduct when their families maintain a predictable pattern.

Your child with ADHD and the rest of the family could benefit from having a set routine. The structure is advantageous for several reasons, including the following:

- Control from the outside: The symptoms of ADHD lead to problems with one's ability to exercise self-control. Because of this, children who have ADHD require a greater number of external controls (also known as structure) to assist them in managing their symptoms.
- Fewer conflicts: Structure can help improve behavior while reducing the stress and fights inside a family. According to the findings of several studies, those who keep to their routines are better able to deal with stress and worry.
- Developing skills and routines: Many children are capable of organizing their chores, timetables, and activities, as well as developing positive habits on their own. On the other hand, due to the functioning of ADHD, this is a task that is significantly more difficult to accomplish when it involves a child.

Structure in the home ensures that every family member adheres to the daily schedule. This benefit extends to all members of the family. A child with ADHD will not feel as though they are being singled out due to this. Children learn to schedule the same amount of time each day to finish their homework or to develop a pattern for going to bed and getting up in the morning. It is possible to make going to school on time the next morning much more achievable by performing straightforward actions the night before, such as having a shower and selecting clothing to wear to school.

Laying the groundwork for success Structure helps children achieve and helps them succeed, fostering self-esteem. If this is not present, children are more likely to perceive that they are disorganized, forgetful, or always running late. Your child will have a better chance of succeeding in life if you establish some exterior constraints in the house. Along the way, you also instill beneficial behaviors and skills in them.

A structure can be introduced into your child's life by providing them with day-to-day routines and a timetable to adhere to. Your child should be able to comprehend the house rules, expectations, and penalties in place, and they should receive positive reinforcement from you. This will assist in creating a predictable atmosphere.

Your child will be better prepared for whatever comes their way in a well-structured environment. Because of this, most children, regardless of whether or not they have attention deficit hyperactivity disorder (ADHD), benefit from having a structure in their lives.

A good analogy for the structure would be scaffolding. In other words, the routines, reminders, and boundaries that you establish, as well as the consistency that you provide, provide the support your child needs to succeed and develop greater competence. Your child's level of self-confidence will increase as a direct consequence of this. Your child will eventually benefit from this by developing abilities that will help them manage and structure their lives as they transition into adulthood.

How To Create A Friendly Schedule

It is essential to devise a routine that can accommodate your child's specific requirements. If you follow a few simple guidelines, you'll be able to create a routine for your child that will be simple for them to stick to, even though your particular routine will be different depending on what works best for your family.

- **Provide limited choices**: Providing your child with restricted options is one method to make their schedule more manageable. As an illustration, rather than inquiring as to what they would like for breakfast, offer them a choice between two or three different alternatives. While still providing structure, this will let them feel more in control of the situation.

- **Be specific**: Be detailed and break down large jobs into smaller ones as much as possible. For instance, rather than referring to "chore time," you may mention the precise tasks that your child will be responsible for, such as "picking up toys," "feeding the dog," or "cleaning the kitchen floor." Breaking up bigger chores into smaller sections will assist in keeping your child's attention and prevent them from feeling overwhelmed.
- **Include visual cues**: Children who have ADHD may benefit from the use of visual cues. You can demonstrate to your child what activities they will participate in throughout the day using a visual schedule. You could represent each activity with words, photos, or even just some simple sketches if you wanted to. Put the schedule somewhere where it can be seen, and make it a habit to go through it with your kid regularly.
- **Make time for movement**: It is generally helpful for children who have ADHD to have multiple opportunities throughout the day to move around. Make sure that you schedule some physical activity every few hours. This can be as straightforward as going for a brief stroll or playing a speedy catch.
- **Be flexible**: Although it is necessary to adhere to a timetable, it is necessary to be adaptable to unforeseen circumstances. Your kid should be allowed to choose whatever activity they want to do next whenever possible, and if they are feeling overwhelmed, they should be allowed to take a break. Depending on what your child needs from day to day, you may need to make adjustments to your routine.

Even if your child pushes back against the routine at first, you must remain steadfast in your adherence to it. This cannot be easy, so it's vital to maintain some degree of flexibility; yet, you shouldn't give up on it too early if you want to succeed.

Your child may feel more in control of their environment and have fewer outbursts or tantrums if you help them create a timetable that accommodates their ADHD. You may assist your child in maintaining focus and staying on task throughout the day by giving them structure and visual clues.

The following ideas can be implemented into your family to give it more structure. You are going to want to modify these suggestions so that they work for your family and the requirements that they have. Don't forget that achieving achievement takes time; thus, you shouldn't give up since it will be worth the wait.

Good Mornings

Parents frequently cite the morning hours as one of the most challenging times to care for their children. We all must leave the house at the designated time. The following are some suggestions for how this can be accomplished:

- Prepare as much as you can the night before, such as taking a bath or shower, choosing outfits and laying them out, packing backpacks and leaving them by the door or in the car, discussing breakfast options, and leaving out whatever does not have to be refrigerated to expedite food preparation, and preparing lunches and placing them in lunch boxes and storing them in the refrigerator.
- Please talk about your child's routine from the moment they first open their eyes, including things like going to the toilet, washing their hands and face, brushing their teeth, getting dressed, and coming downstairs for breakfast, among other things.
- Check on your kid to see how they are doing while getting dressed, and be sure to offer praise whenever appropriate.
- If your kid is in the car or on the school bus and wants to use his phone or read a book, you have to make them buckle up before allowing them to do any of those things.

After School

Let's avoid arguing about the schoolwork and get it done already!

This is a time of day when a child's capacity to self-regulate is called upon, and for the majority of children who have ADHD, it is a genuine struggle, especially after putting in a whole day's worth of effort in academics, emotions, and behavioral management. To increase your output, give some of these strategies a shot:

Provide wholesome food, and then use a timer to determine when snack time should end.

- Maintaining a set beginning time for homework helps establish a habit of completing assignments.
- Do not leave your child unattended, and do not wander off. Remain close by. Many children who have ADHD can maintain their focus better when an adult is around or when they are working alongside an adult.
- If you notice that your child is becoming overwhelmed, encourage them to do a portion of the project at once.

- If you have lengthy assignments, you can make them look more manageable by blocking off part of the page or folding it in half.
- Have your child do a portion of the work, then have them take a little break, and then have them complete the balance of the assignment.
- When trying to block out other noises in the house, it could be good to play some soothing music or white noise in the background.
- Have a conversation with your child about an enjoyable activity that they can do when they have finished their schoolwork before they start. This could motivate your child to complete the assignments they have been given for homework effectively.

Dinners Ready

As a working mother, I know how challenging it can be to get everyone to sit down to supper simultaneously.

It is crucial to make an effort to maintain a consistent dinnertime schedule, regardless of whether you prepare meals at home or order food to be delivered. This is an opportunity for family members to spend time with one another and build stronger bonds.

One of the activities we all look forward to doing together as a family is going around the table and taking turns talking about the positive and negative aspects of the day they have had. During this conversation, several incredibly useful learning opportunities will present themselves, and it will be an excellent opportunity to learn about everyone's recent activities.

Don't forget to ask your children's assistance in setting the table, clearing it afterward, putting away the food, and cleaning the dishes by hand or loading them into the dishwasher. Have a nice meal!

Goodnight

It is just as vital to get a good night's sleep as to eat well and exercise regularly.

Children with attention deficit hyperactivity disorder (ADHD) often resist going to sleep because they find it uninteresting. After all, there is still much work to be done! The following are some ideas that, if tried, can help one feel more relaxed and at ease:

Make it a point to put your child to bed at approximately the same time each night.

- Provide guests with a wholesome and light snack (e.g., rice cake with a small amount of almond butter, jam, or avocado).
- Read to your child or read aloud to them.

- You and your child could participate in a mindful activity or meditate together.
- Have a tender good night routine, such as giving hugs, reading a poem, or praying before bedtime.

On not one but two levels, life is improved by having routines. They contribute to an increase in the effectiveness and the general functioning of daily life. Even though it is not always apparent, children crave and need routines. Kids benefit from a structure in their lives, provided by a routine they can count on. By constructing one, you are sending a signal that says, "This is the way things are done here." Your child can concentrate on one task at a time if you establish routines that make daily duties more doable.

In addition, the psychological well-being of the complete household will improve after you establish a routine and stick to it. When there is less drama about when you'll eat supper and where you'll settle down to complete homework, everyone in the household experiences less stress. This includes the parents as well as the children.

The result is a calmer home environment, leading to closer family ties. The rituals that everyone in the family participates in help bind the family members closer together (Anna sets the table, and Brian clears the dishes). The message is that we are a family that eats together, a family that reads together, and a family that sets up regular times for homework and other tasks that are continuing.

Maintaining a planned lifestyle in this day of nonstop activity might appear tough. Everyone is trying to balance their various commitments, such as work, school, extracurricular activities, recreation, music classes, basketball practice, etc. However, precisely in such circumstances, the structure becomes crucial. The benefits of doing so include increased productivity in your child, improved health, and stronger bonds within the family.

When there are predictable routines in the home, children of all ages, including infants and preschoolers, have better overall health and are better able to self-regulate their behavior, according to a review of psychological research spanning the past 30 years just published in a Journal of Family Psychology.

For routines to be efficient, there must be dedication and consistency on the part of all of the adults in the family. It is best to begin establishing routines for children when they are still small and continue doing so as they age; nevertheless, it is never too late to begin. Most importantly, do not give up.

Below are some tips and sample routines to assist you in getting started. You will want to adjust them to align with your child's age and maturity level, the particular behaviors you are attempting to correct, and the character and requirements of your family. Remember that success takes time, perhaps months or even years, as you develop your habits. However, the advantages will remain for the rest of one's life.

7:00 a.m. Tickle your child out of bed. (A little happy energy can get her up and move quickly.)

7:05 a.m. Get ready: Post a list and have your child stick to it.

Wash face.
Comb hair.
Get dressed. (Clothes are laid out the night before.) Check to see how your child is doing, but let her follow the list and do it for herself.

7:20 a.m. Breakfast time: Offer two healthy but appealing choices, max. You want her to spend her time eating, not pining over Lucky Charms.

7:45 a.m. Brush your teeth—together. Being with her can speed things up and insure good hygiene.

7:55 a.m. Zip, tie, and layer up. Keeping shoes and gloves by the front door spares you the hide-and-seek.

8:00 a.m. Out you go.

Sample Homework Routine

3:00 p.m. Have a snack and unwind from school.

3:30 p.m. Settle your child at his regular homework spot; be sure all tools are available (pencils, paper, calculator, reference books, etc.).

3:35 – 4:30 p.m. Your child does homework; you stay around to answer questions and monitor breaks (stretch, bathroom, drink).

4:25 p.m. Check his work and calmly review anything he should edit (but don't do it for him). Offer specific praise for good work.

Sample Dinner Routine

6:00 p.m. Parent(s) starts food prep. Organize preparation so that you can avoid the delay of mealtime.

6:15 p.m. Kids set the table. Give them specific tasks to instill a sense of responsibility.

6:30 p.m. Kids pour the beverages.

6:45 p.m. Parent(s) brings the food out to the table.

7:00 p.m. Dinner is served. For mealtime talk, try this: Go around the table—once or more—and have each person share one good thing about their day.

7:30 p.m. Kids clear the table. Parent(s) loads the dishwasher.
Sample Bedtime Routine

8:00 p.m. Let him relax in the tub. You can read to him, or he can read to himself. Beyond cleanliness, a bath can help a child mellow out at day's end.

8:20 p.m. Three-part routine: dry off, brush teeth, and pee. You don't want to hear, "Mom, I have to go to the bathroom!" five minutes after you say goodnight.

8:30 p.m. Get into PJs and clean up toys to set a scenario for nighttime, not playtime.

8:40 p.m. Read together.

8:55 p.m. Your child gets into bed. Do your nighttime routine: Talk a little about the day, compliment your child on the things he did well, and say your ritual goodnight — "I love you to the moon and back again. Don't let the bedbugs bite."

HOW TO PREPARE YOUR CHILD FOR ACADEMIC SUCCESS

Problems with attention, the ability to regulate one's impulses, and hyperactivity are the hallmarks of the condition known as attention deficit hyperactivity disorder (ADHD). It is common for symptoms to appear in childhood, although a diagnosis might not be made until puberty or age.

Once children with ADHD start school, their challenges, such as having trouble paying attention, may become more obvious. As a result of this, parents and teachers will need to collaborate to assist children in learning how to manage the symptoms of ADHD.

It is essential to consider the requirements of your child who has attention deficit hyperactivity disorder (ADHD) when getting ready for the back-to-school season (ADHD).

This neurodevelopmental disease is characterized by inattention and impulsivity, which can make it challenging to focus, follow directions, and complete assignments at school. Your child will likely have a more positive experience overall if you take the time to plan and complete these tasks before they start or return to school.

Contact Your Child's Teacher

It is possible for parents of children diagnosed with ADHD to enhance their children's educational outcomes by actively participating in their children's educational process.

It is important to discuss any concerns you might have with the teacher(s) of your kid at the beginning of the school year, regardless of whether or not your child receives formal accommodations at school. Instead of addressing them during the open house, when they are most likely engaged in conversation with numerous families, see if you can schedule an online or in-person meeting after school to discuss the matter.

In addition, it is possible that your child's school does not offer daily physical education programs. It is a good idea to inquire with your child's teacher whether they provide "movement breaks" at certain points throughout the school day so that your child can release excess energy and concentrate more effectively while learning.

Your child may also benefit from sitting in the front of the classroom, closest to their teacher, from assisting in reducing the number of distractions in the learning environment. Your child may be eligible for additional testing time or other adjustments, depending on the individual education program (IEP) or section 504 plan that they have.

Help Organize School Materials

It is possible for parents of children diagnosed with ADHD to enhance their children's educational outcomes by actively participating in their children's educational process.

It is important to discuss any concerns you might have with the teacher(s) of your kid at the beginning of the school year, regardless of whether or not your child receives formal accommodations at school. Instead of addressing them during the open house, when they are most likely engaged in conversation with numerous families, see if you can schedule an online or in-person meeting after school to discuss the matter.

In addition, it is possible that your child's school does not offer daily physical education programs. It is a good idea to inquire with your child's teacher whether they provide "movement breaks" at certain points throughout the school day so that your child can release excess energy and concentrate more effectively while learning.

Your child may also benefit from sitting in the front of the classroom, closest to their teacher, from assisting in reducing the number of distractions in the learning environment. Your child may be eligible for additional testing time or other adjustments, depending on the individual education program (IEP) or section 504 plan that they have.

Back-Up Items

Multiple easily misplaced products will also help you avoid the morning (afternoon and evening) rush. Consider some items that are most likely to be misplaced: Invest in more socks if you find that you are losing them at an alarming rate. If they are running late because of their sneaky shoes (or their keys, gloves, caps, or transport fares), having backups on hand will allow them to get out the door on time.

Head Of Class

Sitting in the front row of the classroom encourages accountability and helps students avoid the distractions (and temptations!) of back-row talk and note-passing. The more challenging it is for children with ADHD to avoid detection and treatment, the better. When children can sit closer to the front of the classroom, their teachers can better observe whether or not they are having difficulty learning the material. This allows you and the instructor to address the issue before it develops into a larger problem.

Help Your Child Establish A School Routine
Your child's ability to refocus when they need to and their capacity for stress and worry are reduced when they have a clear schedule.
You might want to consider writing down the schedule with your child on a large piece of paper, a calendar, or a board and then hanging it on a wall, placing it on the refrigerator, or placing it somewhere else in a common location so that your child can readily refer to it.
Aside from the hours that your child is in school, it would help if you thought about establishing distinct times for the following:
- Daily activities include waking up and getting ready, therapy sessions after school, and extracurricular activities.
- Time for either tutoring or homework, or both, at regular intervals.
- A regular hour for going to bed.

It is also beneficial to go through this routine for a few days of practice before the start of the school year.

Set Up A Homework Routine
When it's time to hit the books, having an organized and regular homework routine will assist both children and their parents in getting their work done without getting into a fight with one another. Create a calm and organized environment for the children to work in where there will be a minimum of interruptions. Don't let them sit in front of a screen during their breaks – they need to get up and move around! Don't forget to give them snacks to maintain their blood sugar levels stable and their concentration high.
Prioritize
Children with ADHD frequently struggle to understand which of their many responsibilities should be prioritized. The use of color coding can be extremely helpful in situations like this one. They should be equipped with highlighters, as well as backup highlighters. A priority level should be assigned to each color. For instance, pink would be considered "high," blue would be considered "mid," and green would be considered "low." They will be able to improve their abilities and better understand what steps to

do at what times with the assistance of a system that has already been built. You might also use applications such as Remember the Milk, which let users input due dates, priority levels, and time estimations for each assignment.

Time Management
Finding a way for children with ADHD to manage their time efficiently is the holy grail of treatment. In addition to calendars, kids can benefit from using task clocks like Focus Booster, which can help them more accurately estimate the time required to complete each activity and alert them when it is time to move on to something else. Timers aren't simply handy for completing homework and chores; they may also be used during longer tests as a reminder to transition between parts and help students make the most of their available time.

Medication Check-In
Children who have been taking their medications regularly but have stopped doing so over the summer should resume doing so in plenty of time before the new school year begins. And when school starts, it's important to pay close attention to how it's working throughout the day (including mornings!) and adjust the schedule so that kids aren't crashing during the last few periods or having mid-math homework meltdowns after school. This will keep them from crashing during the last few periods or having meltdowns after school.

Exercise And Relaxation Techniques
Your child may become worn out during the school week due to the additional necessary concentration. Outside of the possibility of activity breaks throughout the school day, regular exercise throughout the week may also assist your child in expanding energy so that they can concentrate better during the school day and on their homework tasks.
It would be best if you tried to squeeze in some additional exercise whenever you can. Playground visits and time spent running around in parks might be beneficial for children of younger ages. You can inspire older children to participate in sports and accompany you on walks as a family.
On the other hand, learning how to relax and manage stress might help your child become more able to concentrate on what they are

doing. Attention training can benefit from techniques such as meditation and other mindfulness activities. You can begin by teaching your child to concentrate on their breathing by having them take a few minutes each day to do it independently.

Make Use Of Tools And Flexible Rules
Students who have ADHD often have a difficult time sitting still. If it is a normal rule in the classroom that pupils must remain seated during the session, a child with ADHD may have an easier time remaining focused on the topic if they are permitted to stand up.
Holding a little "Koosh Ball" or something tactile to manipulate (like Silly Putty) provides a little stimulation for children who tend to fidget without interrupting the educational environment.
Chewing gum may help some students focus better, according to the findings of some studies; however, these findings have not been replicated by other researchers. Additionally, pupils are not permitted to chew gum in many educational settings.

Don't Overload Them
When dealing with a child who has ADHD and has a tendency to feel overwhelmed, reducing the total amount of work that needs to be done by dividing it into smaller pieces can be helpful.
By providing clear and concise directions in either one or two stages, teachers can assist students in avoiding the feeling of being overwhelmed by information. Children who have ADHD may also have difficulties sleeping, which can hurt their conduct as well as their capacity to pay attention in class.
Students typically feel "fresher" and less weary earlier in the day; nevertheless, adolescents and college students are more prone to have difficulty with early classes. It is also not unheard of for children to experience a little of a letdown after lunchtime.
If it is at all possible, you should make plans to have the students in your class work on the academic subjects and tasks that are the most challenging while they are at their most attentive and engaged.

Encourage Support
Children diagnosed with ADHD may require additional assistance from a classroom aid; however, faculty members are not always available. Similarly, it's possible that students with ADHD don't have access to the academic assistance resources they need.

Even when a child receives one-on-one assistance from an adult, it is occasionally beneficial to make arrangements for the child to have support from their peers. Both children can have a positive learning experience if one student with ADHD is paired with another student who is mature, kind, and eager to help. Encouragement, assistance staying on task or refocusing after being sidetracked, and providing reminders are all things that a child's "study buddy" can do for them.

Working with another student can assist a child who struggles with attention deficit hyperactivity disorder (ADHD) in improving their social skills and the quality of their connections with their classmates. Both of these areas can be challenging for children who have ADHD.

Maintain Positive Reinforcement
In addition to any behavioral tactics, your kid may get at school as part of an Individualized Education Program (IEP) or a Section 504 plan, you should also use positive reinforcement and feedback at home as frequently as possible. It is possible that your child would gain more from receiving comments regarding their ability to focus and complete their assignments than receiving grades.

It is not unheard of for any child, regardless of whether or not they have been diagnosed with ADHD, to experience feelings of being overwhelmed at some point during the academic year. You may assist in lowering your child's stress level by maintaining their schedule, but you should also be on the lookout for clear indicators that your child requires a break from normal activities.

Your commitment to meeting your child's mental and emotional needs on an ongoing basis will, in the long run, help them do better in other aspects of their lives, including in school.

A kid or adolescent suffering from attention deficit hyperactivity disorder may find the classroom to be an environment that is both disorienting and overwhelming (ADHD). Because of the continual presence of sensory overloads, such as background noises, talkative classmates, and lecturing teachers, it can be challenging for children with ADHD to maintain attention, follow directions, and finish homework.

It is a fact that children who have ADHD and their parents who desire to assist them may experience difficulty in academic settings. Children who have attention deficit hyperactivity disorder (ADHD) are more likely to struggle academically than their peers who do not have ADHD. Despite this, children who have ADHD do have a chance of excelling academically, particularly if they have a solid support system that includes not just their parents and teachers but also their classmates and school counselor.

The children diagnosed with ADHD do not all respond the same way to treatment or have the same needs. While a child may benefit from using a checklist, there is no guarantee that this will be the case for all children. Because each child is unique, finding a solution that will work for all of them is impossible.

Talk To The Teacher About Your Child

For some children, the greatest challenge is learning to maintain control of their bodies in an environment that encourages them to sit for extended periods. For some people, the most difficult challenge is blocking out distracting sounds and activities while attempting to zero in on an issue requiring sustained attention and focus, such as a math problem, a science experiment, or a test question. Others have difficulty concentrating on a single task because they have trouble concentrating on multiple tasks simultaneously. Many children with high IQs also have attention deficit hyperactivity disorder (ADHD), which causes their thoughts and ideas to race ahead of the teacher's words. As a result, the situation may leave the individual feeling frustrated and even hopeless, especially if the other pupils in the class remain firmly focused on a slow information-collection process. Because of these obstacles, the current educational environment and methods of instruction need to be modified.

Request For Accommodation That Fits The Child's Learning Style

Once your team has identified what will assist your child in advancing academically, ensure that the school puts modifications in place to assist your child in retaining the information that is being taught to them. For instance, how recent information is communicated to the audience can make a difference.

Students may find that audio, video, or digital content is more engaging and effective than traditional textbooks. Hearing passages from books or questions from exams read aloud to them is helpful to certain people. Others do best when they are allowed to complete their tasks verbally rather than having them handed to them in writing form or when they are provided with a computer to compose their comments.

Consider the possibility of making adjustments to your child's schedule, such as permitting more frequent breaks, giving them a few extra minutes to accomplish assignments, or administering assessments at certain times of the day.

Focus On The Physical Environment

The child's placement inside the classroom can decide how successfully an ADHD student navigates their school day. Mazza points out that there are ways to position children within a classroom so they can pay attention to what is happening around them. "Perhaps they should be seated at the very front, or perhaps they should be seated at a table with no more than three other children." How the space is laid out is of the utmost significance.

Consider the atmosphere while testing: Is it possible to take a test in a more peaceful environment? Where are there only a handful of people? whereas making use of exercise chair bands or other sensory tools for active legs or hands?

Similarly, you should do your best to eliminate as many potential sources of distraction as possible from the environment in which your child studies at home. While studying, you should refrain from checking your email and social media and turn off any notifications that may appear on your phone or other devices.

Develop Tools To Ease Transition

The child's placement inside the classroom can decide how successfully an ADHD student navigates their school day. Mazza points out that there are ways to position children within a classroom so they can pay attention to what is happening around them. "Perhaps they should be seated at the very front, or perhaps they should be seated at a table with no more than three other children." How the space is laid out is of the utmost significance.

Consider the atmosphere while testing: Is it possible to take a test in a more peaceful environment? Where there are only a handful of people? whereas making use of exercise chair bands or other sensory tools for active legs or hands?

Similarly, you should do your best to eliminate as many potential sources of distraction as possible from the environment in which your child studies at home. While studying, you should refrain from checking your email and social media and turn off any notifications that may appear on your phone or other devices.

CONCLUSION

My intention is not to negatively impact these disadvantaged children here. As a result of their inability to exercise self-control, individuals are referred to mental health professionals for treatment. These professionals may include psychologists or psychiatrists. Everyone who has been through anything similar or presently going through something similar is aware of how torturous something like this can be.

In my experience, treating a child with ADHD requires treating the entire family. During my career, I have had the opportunity to assist many families dealing with this issue while their child was receiving treatment from a child psychologist. The goal of therapy for the family was not and is not to engage in bitter griping about the child; rather, it is to acquire particular behavioral methods to manage with the child while providing support to one another rather than engaging in blame-shifting with one another. In addition to this, parents must learn to pay attention to and pay heed to the requirements of their children's other siblings.

Family therapy also focuses on education regarding the disease in question, to prevent parents from blaming themselves for what has occurred to their child. Hope is also essential since many parents wrongly feel their child with ADHD is destined to live the rest of their life with a disability. People who have Attention Deficit Hyperactivity Disorder (ADHD) can go on to live fruitful and happy lives after they figure out how to manage the symptoms of their condition and make the most of the unique abilities that come with having ADHD.

Suppose you are in this scenario and have a child with Attention Deficit Hyperactivity Disorder (ADHD). In that case, you must get help for the child, yourself, and the rest of your family.

Made in United States
Troutdale, OR
06/28/2023

10852901R00077